BREAKING

THROUGH

THE UNTOUCHABLE

DISEASES

By Gerald Green

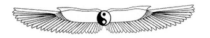

SAGAX Publishing
2008

Published by SAGAX Publishing
P O Box 106
MONMOUTH
NP25 9AB, UK

Copyright © Gerald Green 2008
ISBN 0-9532407-8-9

A catalogue record for this book is available from the British library

Gerald Green's right to be identified as the author of this work has been asserted by him in accordance with the Copyright, Designs and Patent Act 1988.

Manufactured and printed in the United Kingdom by Lightning Source Inc.

Foreword

In 1991, I found *Shangri La. After decades of fast living, poor eating and generally not looking after myself, I became very ill. I was facing a lifetime on steroids after I was misdiagnosed with Crohn's disease.

The tabloids printed an article stating I was on my last legs and I received hundreds of letters of support. Gerald sent a letter that would lead to my full recovery. He educated me all about organic food and the pesticides that are used in farming, explained how chemicals in our food can damage our immune systems and showed me how to heal myself. This was the start of my organic journey and it has become my passion and my work.

Gerald takes a straightforward approach toward the amazing benefits of good food and its incredible healing powers. His inspiring passion and motivated quest to cure auto-immune diseases is unstoppable.

He has become a mentor, a constant source of advice and a recommendation for many of my friends and family.

This book will walk you towards *Shangri La, and I strongly suggest you let it take you on your way. Thanks Gerald for everything you have done.

2008

*Shangri La is the name of Gerald Green's house

Notice

The advice given in this book is based on the author's experience with many hundred's of patients. However it is not intended to provide medical advice or replace the advice of a physician for either medical treatment or the use of the diets within. Always seek advice from your medical practitioner first.

This book is published for the express purpose of sharing educational information, scientific research and personal truth gathered from the research, studies and experiences of the author.

Readers are advised to consult their own doctors or qualified health care professionals regarding the treatment of their medical problems. If readers are taking prescriptions, medications or are pregnant, they should not take themselves off medication to start supplementation without the proper supervision of their physician.

Neither the author nor the publisher takes any responsibility for possible consequences from any treatment, action or preparation for use or mis-use of the herbal medication or diets to any person reading or following the information in this book.

<u>Acknowledgements</u>

Most of what I have achieved has been completely on my own but I would like to thank Chris Woolams of the Icon Network and Philip Day who are men in my type of groove. I would also like to thank Karin Taylor and Pam Blowers, two ladies I taught who could assimilate what I wanted to achieve and they are both brilliant. Not too many could understand what I wanted to convey but they did. But then applied immunology as it really is, as opposed to how orthodoxy would have us believe, is easily the most fascinating subject in the world. He or she who can understand true immunology should be able to take almost any disease apart save genetic and not be long about it.

I would also like to thank Keith Foster, one of my recent patients who following treatment for a nasty gut disease, was so impressed with my work that he encouraged and helped me to get this book published before my death and took my rough written script and had it typed for me.

Finally I would like to thank my daughter Evelyn who has, as with all my other works, vetted and reworded some of my over-passionate opinions of the pharma-medical network.

Contents

INTRODUCTION

You will read in this book how I came to understand the importance of herbal remedies and diet at the age of 45 years. Having found little relief from orthodox treatments, I started to learn the power of herbs and how to use them, firstly for my own salvation and then for many hundreds of other poor sufferers who have come to me to gain relief from some of the world's worst diseases.

Most major auto-immune diseases have one thing in common: when they have been treated by orthodox Candida-inducing drugs like the antibiotic-orientated drugs used for Crohn's and ulcerative-colitis, immuno-suppressives, even chemo-drugs, all of which kill off the good bowel bugs that in nature keep Candida in control, then they will find all or most beneficial medicinal effects will be masked out, causing less or no control of whatever auto-immune disease they were trying to treat.

My work as a herbalist and immunologist is not really work at all because it's a passion to relieve so much unnecessary misery caused through either misunderstanding or no real understanding at all of these dreadful diseases. I realise as I grow old that this state of affairs has been going on for donkey's years and unless something radical is done, it will continue to infinity and I hope this book will bring this dreadful legacy to an end.

During my time in herbalism, I have written 3 booklets relative to the world's worst diseases:

'Inflammatory Bowel Disease – Collectively known as Crohn's Disease and Ulcerative Colitis' (1985 - with notes on all other gut diseases)

'Multiple Sclerosis – Beaten Against all the Odds' (1995)

'How to Change your Bodily Environment to Beat Cancer' (2004)

This book is a summary of all three of my booklets and also goes on to discuss other serious diseases and illnesses that I have been able to successfully treat.

CHAPTER 1

<u>Auto-Immune Diseases</u>

It is vital to explain at the start, how to cut auto-immune diseases to pieces, and not disadvantage the patient as can happen under orthodox treatments. This group of truly awful diseases are then almost as easy to tackle as any others if a few basic principles are remembered.

The whole group of auto-immune diseases are in fact all one and the same disease mechanism, but with obvious different epicentres of immunological attack which gives them their respective names like, for instance, Crohn's disease and similar ulcerative-colitis (the two worst non-malignant gut diseases in the world). Then there is the untouchable multiple sclerosis (MS) for which orthodox medicine can do little save palliative care and the diagnosis which can take years and when they do get one for this horrible neurological disease, it's like a "death sentence". Then there's rheumatoid arthritis which attacks the joints often causing awful pain and crippling after years of suffering. Unlike most other auto-immune diseases rheumatoid arthritis rarely kills, though some have died because of the strong side-effects of the orthodox pain-killing drugs used which are often harsh on the gut system and can cause internal bleeding.

Some auto-immune diseases are what I call "multiples" and these attack more than one area and are amongst the most dangerous of the lot like systemic lupus (SLE) that can attack the joints, the skin, vascular system, the kidneys, indeed several vital organs. Another is Sjogren's syndrome when the wrongly programmed immune system attacks the secretory glands which supply the joints with lubricating fluid, the mouth and digestive system with saliva and the eyes with essential tears. These then tend to dry up causing great suffering re painful joints, makes the mouth as "dry as sandpaper" affecting digestion, swallowing food, sleep and the teeth go bad re no protection from saliva and finally the eyes are sore through lack of lubricating tears which causes intense suffering.

There are several more auto-immune diseases with names like Hashimoto's disease and Graves disease where the thyroid and the parts this governs are attacked, often giving multiple symptoms relative to what this master gland controls. Indeed if ever you come across a disease of unknown origin (that's not genetic) it's almost certainly in my auto-immune group.

I am certain I know the actual cause and origin of auto-immune disease and you work out who you think is right. Orthodox bodies don't like, (possibly because of their association with the chemical and pharmaceutical industry) chemicals blamed in any way relative to disease, but I have no such qualms. We are subjected to thousands of chemicals produced as additives in our food, drink, insecticides, fungicides and sheep and cattle dips. They are all supposed to be "all right" for human consumption, but as they are made by huge multi-national cartels who can influence governments and other bodies like the Common Market to let "iffy" items continue in use, is it any wonder a wide spectrum of awful diseases are increasing massively in numbers over say the last fifty years especially cancers and auto-immune diseases?

What exactly are auto-immune diseases? No-one to date has given a satisfactory answer to this question and all orthodoxy says is diseases of unknown origins and therefore no specific treatment can be given, except the use of their latter day "leeches" antibiotic-orientated drugs, steroids, immuno-suppressives and even chemotherapy drugs. These then kill off the approximately two pounds in weight of very highly beneficial bugs, that in nature keep the absolute key player in any serious disease namely Candida in control.

Candida

Candida in its normal friendly yeast format is part of the good bugs food source and is as a result an ever growing organism. The good bugs help us digest our food and release all the goodies we need for everyday life. They kill bad bugs, indeed they are vital for our well being and are meant to be in our gut system. However, as you will learn, Candida can be, because of the drugs mentioned above, a Jekyll and Hyde character in that it is given to us in its friendly yeast form to feed billions of highly beneficial digestive bugs necessary for every day healthy living. However, with all these bugs killed off by the very drugs used for auto-immune or any serious disease, there is obviously nothing now to feed on this once friendly ever growing organism. Therefore it grows out of control and we see Candida change from its friendly yeast format into a very unfriendly parasitic fungus.

How can this former food of the good digestive bugs become a key player in these diseases?

Candida now in, as explained, its unfriendly parasitic format spreads as all fungi do by means of whitish threads called mycelium (similar to those one sees in moulds). Although they only look a bit like spiders webs in thickness they can and do puncture almost anything organic and can puncture the bowel wall with ease causing the well known "leaky-gut" syndrome in the colon or large bowel. Why does Candida want to get into the bloodstream in the first place? Candida being a living organism has likes and dislikes as to what it ingests like us. It loves, above all else, sugar but also yeast, and cows milk and all its products. So once in the bloodstream or vascular system you don't have to be Albert Einstein to realise where Candida gets its sugar from. Yes of course the blood sugar on which our energy depends and hence why almost all very ill patients feel fatigued. That's not all because when it's parasitized the blood sugar, it converts this into alcohol, which in turn attacks the liver and the patient often has a "hang over" wakening. Does it ring a bell?

Coming back to Candida's puncturing the bowel wall causing the leaky-gut syndrome. This is a major factor in any auto-immune disease and here's why. All auto-immune patients have a poor digestive enzyme output, so if, for instance, they drank or ate products made from a big animal with four stomachs, namely a cow, they will most likely not digest it at all. As a result it would arrive in the large bowel unchanged from how the patient ingested it. Protein from these cows milk products could easily pass through the bowel wall punctures made by Candida into the bloodstream.

The body's immune system has to stop this protein from flooding the bloodstream, but in so doing often creates dietary allergens that on ingestion then trigger the symptoms of the auto-immune disease relative, eg: gut symptoms for Crohn's disease or neurological for MS and so on. Depending on how often the patient ingests these allergens, can cause the wild fluctuations of symptoms one gets with all auto-immune diseases. I have already mentioned cows milk and products are a very common allergen, however, in exactly the same way many other dietary allergens can be created from leaking of dietary item proteins through the bowel wall. This is why there are often six to eight dietary triggers to auto-immune symptoms.

CHAPTER 2

The Immune System

Now, without overloading the brain, I will try and give a basic simplified version on the complex subject of immunology. I refer to simple applied immunology as everything that runs really well to maximum efficiency as having a rank and file. So if we look at a military army as a way of explaining the immune system, remembering we have millions of immunological "soldiers" that look after the well being of our bodies called lymphocytes, then there is no better way. Armies, as most people know, have generals, normal officers and private soldiers.

So we will call the T cell lymphocytes the generals as they give the orders to attack the enemy constantly attacking us. Then we have the B cell lymphocytes generated in the bone marrow and hence why it's called a B cell, which do most of the killing of the multiple enemies that attack us, these being the officer class. Finally, we have the B cell antibodies which kill viruses like colds and flu and these are the lowest rank, namely the private soldiers and collectively they are called regiments.

Each of these regiments is given a vital part of our bodies or systems of our bodies to look after, all under the jurisdiction of the general T cells with a communication circuit that would make anything we humans achieve look very puny indeed. Thus we are protected from any attack at any time from any quarter. So what goes wrong in auto-immune diseases? We are subjected to hundreds, if not thousands, of chemicals in our every day food. However, I believe one particular chemical used first as a German WW1 nerve gas, namely organo-phosphorus is the main culprit for it is used as an insecticide on a lot of our food and sheep are dipped in it as an anti-scab method, while cattle are treated against warble fly in a similar way.

Most of our food, unless organic, is therefore contaminated with this deadly chemical which we are told is "safe for human consumption", but what about those with a fragility in their immune systems possibly compromised by one thousand and one other chemicals used on us? What I am certain of, and it's the only way auto-immune disease can be logically explained, is that because of these chemicals the general-like T cells mis-programme usually just one of the multiple regiments of officer-like B cells protecting all of our vital organs and body systems. Now mis-programmed by the T cells instead of protecting our vitals, the B cell regiment attacks usually just one vital part of our bodies like, for instance, if it was the regiment formerly protecting the lower small bowel, but now attacking it it's called Crohn's disease. If the regiment was relative to the large bowel it's called ulcerative-colitis, collectively called inflammatory bowel disease and the above are the two worst non-malignant gut diseases in the world. When you want to move a limb, or even blink an eye the message from your brain is as electrical as your house wiring circuit and in exactly the same way your personal "wiring" (your nerves) are insulated by the myelin sheath.

Can you imagine what happens when the regiment of lymphocytes formerly protecting the insulatory myelin sheath, now wrongly programmed attack it causing the electrical charges from the brain to short circuit resulting in malfunction, or no function at all – then this auto-immune disease is called multiple sclerosis, a truly horrible neurological disease that maims, cripples and sadly in primary progressive MS often kills. Orthodox treatments are mostly powerless against this disease save to give palliative treatment.

If the wrongly programmed regiment was formerly protecting the joints but now attacks them, it's called rheumatoid arthritis (which must not be confused with osteoarthritis which is wear and tear) where even young children can have joint replacement operations showing just how destructive these mis-programmed lymphocytes can be.

If the attack is against the thyroid gland, it's called Hashimoto's disease. Sometimes more than one regiment of lymphocytes are wrongly programmed and these are obviously the worst of the lot of auto-immune diseases with names like systemic lupus which attacks nine females to one male. Here usually five regiments become wrongly programmed. These include the skin, vascular system, joints, kidney and several other vital organ regiments numbering to some ten all told, of which usually any one patient suffers from five of these. This then obviously is the most dangerous of the lot. Sometimes the lupus patient gets a rash over the bridge of the nose that looks a bit like a wolf's head and the Latin name for wolf is lupus, hence its name.

Another multiple auto-immune disease is **Sjogren's syndrome**, which although not as dangerous as lupus is, in my opinion, a really devilish disease in that it again attacks nine women to one man. There are usually three regiments attacking what they formerly protected but in this case they attack the secretory glands that supply our eyes with lubricating tears, our mouths with lubricating and digestive saliva, and our joints with again lubricating synovial fluid causing obvious joint pain called immunological arthritis.

Can you imagine what it would be like to have dry, sore, gritty eyes, a mouth that's parched and so dry you can hardly swallow and throat like sandpaper, plus poor and often painful digestion, not to mention joint pain. Because this devilish disease attacks mostly women often doctors take many years to diagnose this as Sjogren's syndrome, often fobbing the ladies off with diagnosis, like "all in the mind" or PMT etc. etc. yet this is the only disease that attacks these three secretory glands and it should be very easy to diagnose when the above symptoms are displayed.

Clare suffered terribly from an 'undiagnosed disease' for nearly two years which a group of top orthodox specialists failed to recognise the fairly classic symptoms of Sjogren's syndrome. When Clare phoned me saying her joints were very painful and her eyes were sore through lack of lubricating tears, and her mouth and throat were dry making eating, digestion and sleeping very difficult, it seemed obvious it was Sjogren's. I used the anti parasitic herb wormwood to wipe out Candida in its parasitic fungal format and my immune ingredient <u>which stops self immunological attack quickly in a low density Candida patient.</u>

The above "Chamber of Horrors" was quickly reduced to near total remission in a few weeks. Also Clare's quality of life has improved to near normal and she is able to work again – almost overnight compared to the timescale suffering under her orthodox "specialists". See letter below from Clare:

"19/12/2005
Dear Mr Green

I came to see you just under a month ago and you kindly spent some time explaining your research and findings with auto-immune problems and cancer.

I went away with a 'trial' as you called it, of your wormwood herbs & immune ingredient. I am so pleased to be able to write and, as you probably suspected, to tell you how much better I'm feeling after just three weeks.

I no longer have: aching joints and muscles, headache, nausea, sleepless nights, dry eyes and mouth, itchy skin, fatigue or pain after eating.

I'm so very grateful! My ears still burn but it's only been 3 weeks!! I feel sure if my problems, even though undiagnosed by the doctors had been left, I would still be waiting for diagnosis and would be a lot worse by now. I really was starting to despair.

I really hope your work gets the recognition it deserves – so many people could be spared a lot of unnecessary treatments.

I would be more than happy for you to give my name and phone number to anyone who wants to double-check the good results your work is doing.

Also I'm now able to work a full week! Thank you.

God Bless

Clare Adams"

In Black's Medical Dictionary under Sjogren's syndrome it says: "<u>treatment is unsatisfactory</u>." I'd say it is, as it is with most auto-immune diseases where often in medical books it says: "Disease of unknown origin", and therefore specific medicines are not usually used, except to use the usual medicines when they don't know the answer like steroids, immuno-suppressives, anti-reject (organs) drugs and sometimes even chemotherapy drugs with awful side effects. These, as already stated, create their own downfall by killing off the good bowel bugs (which would normally keep Candida in control being its food source). However out of control in its parasitic fungal format because of the above drugs Candida has the ability to cause "101" problems the worst of which are:-

1.   <u>To mask out medicinal effect.</u>

2.   <u>To create dietary allergens that on ingestion are then liable to trigger the symptoms of the relevant auto-immune disease.</u>

3.   <u>Until these dietary allergens are eliminated by my exclusion dietary method (explained further on), these are as equally medicinally masking as drug-induced Candida that created these symptom triggering allergens in the first place.</u>

This then is exactly what makes the auto-immune group of diseases the title of this book "Breaking Through The Untouchable Diseases"

CHAPTER 3

My Introduction and Progression into Herbalism Ulcerative Colitis and Crohn's Disease

I can remember when I first tried to take on some of the world's worst diseases, having been very successful by saving my own life from bronchial asthma and emphysema in '76, after being in Brompton Hospital, which sorted me out. I altered my herbal lung formula to use on a seven-year duration duodenal ulcer which often put me in absolute agony and my doctor prescribed pain killers that did nothing at all to cure it. Again I was successful first time curing this devilish ulcer in four and a half weeks.

Then I read a booklet left on the train seat from the National Association of Colitis and Crohn's disease. The first part of which was written by a gastroenterologist showing many ways of having your inside removed with stomach and waste product bags. I thought to myself this must "cheer up" the members no end! Then there was a lot about raising money for "research" which I found out later had achieved little for

18

these people with this terrible disease. Then finally, I read in the back of this NACC booklet two pages on Memoriam on the poor members who had died of these world's worst non-malignant bowel diseases. I thought to myself "I'll crack these awful diseases or die in the attempt!"

People who know me will tell you I'm like this with anything really bad. So how do I contact these poor souls? Well in these disease charity pamphlets there is a pen-friend section so I wrote to all five of them explaining how successful I was in curing my duodenal ulcer and would like to have a go helping them. In my blind enthusiasm I expected them to reply by return of post. Five weeks later a Mrs S. from Lewes replied saying she had ulcerative colitis and although her husband thought me a "crank", she was in dire straights and lined up for a colostomy if I failed to help her.

Teutonic to a fault I thought nothing like being "thrown in the deep end of the pool" so I sent Mrs S her herbal medicine in powder for her to make up in liquid format and to take four wine-glassfuls a day. It annihilated her every symptom and the colostomy operation was cancelled! To say I was "over the moon" would have been the understatement of the year and Mrs S. 100% relief remission was sustained.

Mrs S. then phoned me to say she had a friend in the NACC with similar Crohn's disease could I do anything? "Oh yes", I replied, "it should be a 'piece of cake' ". "Pride, as they say, comes before the fall" because I sent off to Mrs S's friend exactly the same herbal formula and instructions called the gut Triple Alliance formula and she phoned me to say it had no beneficial effect at all! I was utterly devastated for how on earth could my formula work so well with a miraculous result on one patient, yet exactly the same formula and instructions failed so miserably on her friend with similar Crohn's disease.

To cut a long story short, the above state of affairs carried on for nearly three years i.e. getting a brilliant result with one patient, nothing with another, or something in between. What I was doing was worthwhile and saved a lot of misery and suffering but I did feel so sorry for those it did not work on. I asked my friends in alternative medicine about this odd scenario and they said, "oh you win some, lose some. " This however was not good enough for me for there simply had to be a scientific reason for what was happening.

The Anti-Candida Diet

Then I received some medical papers from America where a medic out there stated that drug-induced Candida could mask out most or all medicinal effects. This news was like a gift from God to me and from now on I used the anti-candida diet (universally disregarded by orthodoxy) on all my patients and for those who did not mind contributing toward their own salvation with the strict diet, remission was their reward nearly every time.

You may look at the list below and feel despondent, but please be assured, it is a small price to pay for what you will GAIN.

After following this diet for a few days, you should notice increased energy, easier movement, better sleep, less digestive problems, in fact, many people report ALL their symptoms disappear, especially when they use the herbs and supplements suggested.

ELIMINATE:

All cows milk and products: butter, cheese, yoghurt, whey - all cow's milk derivatives such as the protein casein and lactose.

Yeast products: Alcohol, bread and all its relatives (soda bread is allowed), marmite, oxo, bovril, vinegars, mushrooms, processed and smoked fish and meats.

Sugar and sugar products: sucrose, honey, fructose, lactose, glucose, dextrose plus any sugar alternatives which contain aspartame or canderal.

Nearly all fruit: overripe fruits are full of sugar and yeast and dried fruits.

High-sugar root vegetables: carrots, parsnips, sweet potatoes, beetroots etc. NB: if you really can't live without potatoes, wean yourself off them slowly and try to end up with one a day.

Carbohydrates: Carbohydrates convert to sugar in the gut so cut out 85%. These are the grains like wheat, oats, barley, rye and rice plus potatoes etc.

Avoid all convenience/junk foods as they contain hidden sugars and undesirable ingredients.

Avoid health supplements or anything else containing lactose, citric acid, sugar, casein yeast or whey.

Avoid crackers, pastries, doughnuts, cakes, pies, muffins cookies and most breads (a little soda bread is ok).
Snacks including crisps, pretzels and popcorn.
White rice, potatoes and corn.

Products made with white flour, such as pasta.
(If you feel you can't cut out potatoes completely, wean yourself off them slowly and try to end up with one a day)

Chick peas, dried beans, lentils, pinto beans, peas. Mushrooms and fungi

Processed meats such as bacon, sausage, ham, salami, bologna, pastrami, hot dogs and smoked fish and farmed salmon and trout.

High-salt foods such as processed meats, fish and in particular smoked fish.

Condiments such as pickles and all shop bought sauces.

Hydrogenated fatty acids and partially hydrogenated fatty acids as contained in some margarines and many processed foods.

Saturated fats from tropical oils such as coconut oil and palm oil.

Saturated fats of any type, especially from meat and meat products.

The following fruit and vegetables in particular are best avoided:

Apricots, bananas, blackberries, grapefruit, grapes, kumquats, passion fruit, peaches, plums, raspberries, strawberries, any melon. Artichokes, asparagus, aubergine, avocado, courgettes, okra, peas, pumpkin, sauerkraut, sugar snap peas, squash.

If you fancied say raspberries, do away with your apple that day and have the equivalent in raspberries.

The list above shows you the foods Candida loves and thrives on. Most of these need to be eliminated from your diet for ever. However, when in remission, asparagus, aubergine, avocado, courgettes, peas raspberries, strawberries and plums can be reintroduced.

GOOD FOOD CHOICES

The foods below have the lowest possible sugar/yeast content and are your best choice. You will notice there are several oils included, this is because certain 'good fats' are vital for health, these are linseed and cod liver oil (Omega 3) and evening primrose oil (Omega 6). The ideal ratio is 3 parts Omega 3 to 1 part of Omega 6. i.e. a dessertspoon of linseed or cod liver oil mixed with a 100mg capsule of evening primrose oil once a day.

Eat plenty of the following foods:

Alfalfa sprouts, bean sprouts, sweet peppers, box choy, green broccoli, brussel sprouts, cabbage, cauliflower, celery, cucumber, endive, fennel, garlic, green beans, greens, hot chilli peppers, kale, lettuce, onions, parsley, radishes, spring onions, spinach, swiss chard, turnips, watercress, swede, celeriac, chicory, kohl rabi, leeks and ginger.

Granose sunflower margarine and Tomor kosher margarine (both these margarines should be available at your local health food shop).

Fats (in moderation)

Avocado oil, fish oil, flaxseed oil, grapeseed oil, hemp oil, olive oil, primrose oil and sunflower oil.

Other good foods

Free range eggs
Fresh fish and seafood (but not farmed salmon or trout) - tinned is ok.
Pork, lamb, veal, poultry: chicken, turkey (particularly skinless white meat) - try to get lean meat.
Game
Brazil nuts (in moderation)
Apricot kernels (in moderation)
Tofu (in moderation)
Quorn (in moderation)
Soy milk/cheeses (in moderation)
Rice milk
sheep's milk, and cheeses (dilute 50/50 with water and it taste's like cow's milk)
Goats milk and cheeses
Sunflower, pumpkin and sesame seeds.

Yeast-less bread = soda bread (look out for added sugars and other undesirable ingredients in commercially produced soda breads) and remember any bread is carbohydrate.

Culinary herbs and spices.

Fruit: have <u>only one</u> apple, pear or kiwi a day or equivalent amount of one apple to say strawberries or raspberries but not both.

Fluids

Try to drink 8 glasses of water each day: the body is 60-70% water, so needs fresh supplies daily for optimal hydration and to help flush out toxins. If you can get into the habit of drinking more water, the benefits are many - you will notice increased energy, better concentration, clearer skin to name but a few. You can to advantage add a half teaspoonful of freshly ground powdered cinnamon 2 x day to these glasses of water. This keeps the blood sugar more stable.

Herbal teas are acceptable and green tea is fine.

As mentioned before, the best alternative to sugar is the herb Stevia which is by far the best alternative sweetener because it is anti-fungal (or if you like anti-Candida). Then I find it has been made illegal by the Common Market to sell it in Britain - hence the American website address.

Naturally I wonder why, especially when you see the fantastic fine physique of the South American Indians who use Stevia to sweeten their jungle fare. Looking into it further, I find this 100% natural herb is also excellent for weight loss, or for those on a low carb diet, and also in the use of diabetes. It makes me wonder if there is just not enough money to be made out of this

100% natural herb from the sugar cartels. Please read the write up on the website I have given you www.nowfoods.com this provides some excellent information on the herb.

The following diet is used by most patients with auto-immune diseases, (however, for cancer it's easier with just the need for the anti-candida diet and the reduction of carbohydrates).

Exclusion Dietary Method

This dietary method is to eliminate candida induced dietary allergens. On an A4 chart the patient selects a given number of good foods choices (ie nothing candida likes) and one drink – say 20 all told which they can pick and choose from. On the left hand edge of this chart vertically as example. In the space on the right of these 20 numbered foods and drink, the chart is made up whereby the patient is allowed on each given day 9 foods and a drink ie 10 items in total and they simply fill in for each day of the week. They can vary their choices each day from the 20 items on the left of the chart however they choose.

Now we have a foolproof method of picking out and eliminating any dietary allergen proven where the patient cuts out in numerical order for 5 days one dietary item. <u>Obviously if the patient gets relief on any given exclusion, that is the allergen or one of them so they eliminate this and replace with a sensible alternative.</u>

They must however continue through to number 20 to ensure that they do not have any other allergens. Then with nothing to mask out the medicinal effect the gut Triple Alliance/whatever of my formula's for auto immune diseases will "cut the relative disease to pieces".

Not every patient has these allergens like Mrs S and Katie (referred to in this book), both ulcerative colitis sufferers who had every awful symptom annihilated in only a few days/two days respectively, but for those who, for reasons given, cannot make fast progress, the dietary chart format is the best way to remission. At remission, the patient gets bonuses. Instead of cutting out one dietary item at a time, they add another sensible item (from the temporary excluded group of dietary items) again for 5 days each and if it does not react on them, they can simply add it to their dietary numbers so eventually building up their dietary numbers to 80% of what they used to ingest prior to whatever auto-immune disease they had. They can then also live in up to 100% relief remission as most of my patients do.

There are lots of other benefits like no drug side effects and being as fit and healthy as any unaffected person – the only difference being that they had to work for this wonderful state of remission.

When in remission (up to 100% relief) from inflammatory bowel disease, you get another bonus for being good with the diet – namely you no longer need the labour intensive delayed release capsules. So in lieu I give you two extra weeks supply of the normal Triple Alliance capsules, extending your treatment time from the initial 5 weeks prior to remission to 7 weeks at no extra cost. These then keep you in remission

<u>Please hang your personal dietary chart in the kitchen and ensure you strictly follow this each day.</u>

PERSONAL DIETARY CHART
FOODS & 1 DRINK

#	Food	MON	TUE
1			
		1	1
2		2	2
		3	3
3		4	4
		5	5
4		6	6
		7	7
5		8	8
		9	9
6		10	10
		WED	**THU**
7		1	1
		2	2
8		3	3
		4	4
9		5	5
		6	6
10		7	7
		8	8
11		9	9
		10	10
12		**FRI**	**SAT**
		1	1
13		2	2
		3	3
14		4	4
		5	5
15		6	6
		7	7
16		8	8
		9	9
17		10	10
		SUN	
18		1	
		2	
19		3	
		4	
20		5	
		6	
		7	
		8	
		9	
		10	

Please also note that auto immune diseases need extra dietary care relative to the disease concerned, and I cover this in detail in my individual booklets mentioned at the beginning of this book.

Now I had truly cracked inflammatory bowel disease as Crohn's disease and ulcerative-colitis are collectively known. It was brilliant being able to end the terrible suffering from two of the world's worst non-malignant gut diseases. Also, where under orthodoxy, a high percentage have major surgery as the norm, this proves conclusively that the very antibiotic sulphur-based drugs eventually procreate their own medicinal masking Candida. This in turn sends the disease out of control leading to this horrific surgery rate.

As time went on I realised my liquid format medicine was rather inconvenient so I encapsulated the herbal powders made from liquorice which has a systemic anti-inflammatory effect in the gut, slippery elm a wonderful healing medicine and finally the very expensive golden seal which is a brilliant anti-inflammatory medicine and called this the gut Triple Alliance formula as stated.

Delay release capsules

The encapsulation of this brilliant formula gave me an idea on how to improve further the medications effect by delay releasing some of these capsules direct into the gut. This was done by coating the gelatine capsules with a special composite wax made from bees wax and a weakening agent (as I found bees wax on its own went straight through the patient to no effect).

Eventually I evolved a delayed release capsule which released in the last part of the small bowel where Crohn's epicentre of attack usually is, while ulcerative-colitis usually attacks the large bowel or colon but the two similar diseases sometimes overlap. I rely on the digestive enzymes from the pancreas to weaken the capsule wall so that by the time it had travelled some seventeen feet of the twenty one feet of small bowel, the highly compressed Triple Alliance formula is released at 100% strength as the capsule wall is broken down right in the epicentre of where immunological attack takes place in inflammatory bowel disease.

Not only that, but on release in the small bowel the highly compressed Triple Alliance formula swells into a ball of anti-inflammatory gel because of the slippery elm it contained and was now like a "heat seeking" missile that could not miss its target and coating the whole bowel wall from this point onward in this anti-inflammatory gel that attacks and keeps attacking, laying in situ on the bowel wall to eliminate inflammation and ulceration that are the hall marks of this awful disease.

So you see it was not just a case of giving convenience to my patients through encapsulation but also applied mechanics re my delayed release capsules, impossible with my original liquid format of the gut Triple Alliance formula.

Its success had to be seen to be believed, but it's very difficult when all major alternative news outlets are banned from gaining publicity. So to partially get over this, I had progress charts printed exactly like those illustrated here where at a glance you could see on the left hand side of the chart the symptoms of the relative disease. Then in column 0 or start of the treatment one can see exactly how this patient was like under the doctor with the simple prefix S for severe, M for moderate and SL for slight against the respective symptoms. Then in weeks 1, 2, 3, & 4 the progress of the patient can easily be followed where the S for severe and M for moderate can clearly be seen to lessen quickly to the word gone where appropriate in the following weeks to very little or nothing by one month's treatment. I think you will agree you can't have anything fairer than this and these are 100% genuine cases - my patients can be contacted for references.

Next are 2 progress charts for Crohn's patients Cassandra and Zoe which show how their symptoms were quickly brought to an end and one very severe ulcerative colitis letter from Katie.

Cassandra

Cassandra's Crohn's disease symptoms as can clearly be seen in column '0' were severe, not to mention being hospitalised three times in two years under orthodox treatment. All of this largely unnecessary awful suffering was brought to a sudden halt in only a few weeks with totally safe herbal medicines (without side effects), and all threatened surgery (suffered by a high percentage of Crohn's sufferers) done away with for a life worth living in up to 100% relief remission

Zoe

In Zoe's progress chart, her dreadful Crohn's symptoms were quickly put into remission by a superior natural medication and simple applied immunology re essential dietary regime.

MONITORING CHART for CROHN'S and ULCERATIVE COLITIS

DAY/DATE 10 – 3 – 07	0	Week 1	Week 2	Week 3	Week 4
Symptoms	S	S	M	SL	Gone
Pain / Colic	S	S	SL	VSL	Gone
Bleeding	S	M	SL	Gone	Gone
Number of bowel movements daily	5-6 at least	5-4	2-3	2	2
Fistulas	V.S	M	SL	Gone	Gone
Number of operations prior to herbal / dietary treatment. Please state which.	A flexi sig and also had my fistulas operation.				
Bowel narrowing	S	M	M	SL	Gone
Nausea and sickness	S	M	SL	SL	SL
Emaciation and weight loss	S	S	S	SL	SL
Associated arthritis	M	SL	SL	Gone	Gone
Associated anaemia	S	SL	None	Gone	Gone
Bloating or distension	S	S	M	SL	SL
Constipation	–	None	None	Gone	Gone
Proctitis	–	None	None	SL None	Gone
Stools formed as opposed to diarrhoea	O	M	M	SL	SL
Areas affected but not normally associated by IBD	Eyes & gums				
Drugs taken, please state;	Prednisolone, Ad Cal D3, no longer required				
Relief given	Stopped diarrhoea quickly & all other symptoms				
Any other symptoms; please state.	K nelrad Tiredness	Still tired old	Still tired	Still tired.	
General opinion of herbal v drug treatment	Absolutely amazed at how quickly the herbal tablets took control of the Crohns				
What was the response from your gastroenterologist upon embarking on this treatment?	Not very positive and insisted I continue being admitted to hospital for Inflivimab infusions.				

Please indicate severity of symptoms prior to treatment in column O, for example:
S = SEVERE   M = MODERATE   SL = SLIGHT
Using this code, continue through the weeks, showing relief or lack of it and write the word GONE where relative.
Week O is the start of treatment, please indicate whether or not symptoms are slight, moderate or severe.

Name	Mrs Cassandra C
Address	
Telephone Number	
Comments;	I would highly recommend these herbal tablets instead of any treatment offered by the NHS.

36

MONITORING CHART for CROHN'S and ULCERATIVE COLITIS

DAY/DATE 18/4/2007. BEGAN	0	Week 1	Week 2	Week 3	Week 4
Symptoms					
Pain / Colic	S	S	M	SL	GONE
Bleeding	SL	GONE	—	—	GONE
Number of bowel movements daily	15+	8	7	2	2
Fistulas	NA		✱ BEGIN TO SLEEP THRU NIGHTS		
Number of operations prior to herbal / dietary treatment. Please state which.	NA - FULL COLONOSCOPY TO DIAGNOSE.				
Bowel narrowing	M	SL	SL	GONE	GONE
Nausea and sickness	S	S	M	SL	GONE.
Emaciation and weight loss	S	S	GAINING	GAINING	STILL.
Associated arthritis	NA	—			
Associated anaemia	NA.				
Bloating or distension	S	S	M	SL GASSY	GONE
Constipation	NA				
Proctitis	NA.				
Stools formed as opposed to diarrhoea	O	SL	SL	MOSTLY FORMED	
Areas affected but not normally associated by IBD	CALCIUM D3 FORTE, ACIDOPHILUS-BIFIDASP. VIT B COMPLEX, V.T C.				
Drugs taken, please state;	PREDNISOLONE 7.5mg 7.5mg Cms. 5mg. 3.75				
Relief given	QUICKLY STOPPED OR CALMED ALL SYMPTOMS				
Any other symptoms; please state. FEVER	EXHAUSTED S-M	WEARY S	TIRED OUT SL	GONE	MUCH BETTER NOW
General opinion of herbal v drug treatment	FEEL THAT THIS IS ACTIVELY HEALING ME DRUGS WERE MERELY SUSPENDING SYMPTOMS				
What was the response from your gastroenterologist upon embarking on this treatment?	SEES CANDIDA AS A SCAPEGOAT BUT WAS GENERALLY POSITIVE. STILL THINKS I SHOULD TAKE LONG TERM IMMUNOMODULATOR EVEN IF WELL.				IF HE WOULD C/OHIM CAUSING THE PROBLEM.

Please indicate severity of symptoms prior to treatment in column O, for example:
S = SEVERE   M = MODERATE   SL = SLIGHT

Using this code, continue through the weeks, showing relief or lack of it and write the word GONE where relative.

Week O is the start of treatment, please indicate whether or not symptoms are slight, moderate or severe.

Name	ZOE K
Address	
	LONDON
Telephone Number	
Comments;	SO HAPPY TO NO LONGER BE CHAINED TO A BATHROOM!

HAD A SEVERE "CANDIDA DIE OFF" ~ 8-10 DAYS IN WITH WORSENING OF ALL SYMPTOMS + MORE INTENSE FEVER + EXHAUSTION BUT SINCE THEN EACH DAY HAS SEEN A SLIGHT IMPROVEMENT FROM THE LAST STILL GETTING USED TO THE SENSATION OF FOOD STAYING IN MY GUT AFTER SO LONG GOING THROUGH TOO FAST! GC CALLED HEXHEIMERS SYNDROME RE KILL OFF OF MEDICAL DRUG INDUCED CANDIDA THE KEY PLAYER IN THIS DISEASE C/O DOCTORS

37

Dear Mr Green,

just a quick note to ask for more 'triple-alliance'. (cheque enclosed)
I am _so_ healthy my muscle tone improves daily, meal times refresh me
rather than leading to malaise and pain.

I feel more confident and _ever_ so thankful to yourself and the God in heaven
who has obviously given your gifts and abilities.

I am in the process of returning to Nursing and I have been able to
tell other Nurses of your remedies one Nurse works in a Rheumatology/Neurology
Outpatients department. She has many Lupus patients with little or no hope.

She is unofficially willing to pass on your name & number to patients
So please send me some info & cards and I'll pass them on!

As for me ironically I may be assigned to surgical wards.
as you know. In my proffessional capacity I am not at liberty to
influence anyone's health choices, but on a personal level if your card sometimes
slipped into patients belongings (who would know the difference).

I hope I will be able to pass on my hopeful experiences without causing
harm to patients or my proffession. I intend to try. Obviously I would
hope you would keep this fact confidential for my sake & others!

Nurses are often more open minded when there are patients who surgery &
medicine hold no hope for!

You have helped me to return to a quality of life which I'd almost
forgotten, I hope that my experiences will help me to be sensitive
& helpful & hopeful towards all my patients.

We are on holiday for all of August (I am house sitting for a friend
while Fred decorates) This would not have been possible before taking
the medicine and altering my diet. Thankyou so much Mr Green
Keep up the good work I want others to experience the joys of
healthy symptom free life without side effects or surgery.

With grattitude & respect

Katie

Katie

Katie had very severe ulcerative colitis which brought to an end her beloved nursing career. However, with my Triple Alliance capsules and essential diets, Katie was <u>symptomless in only 2 days</u> (my personal record, although 4 days to total relief is not unusual). She was now able to return to her nursing.

CHAPTER 4

Multiple Sclerosis

Now I could knock out an immunological IBD flare in a few days, impossible by any other method. This meant that this otherwise once difficult disease to treat was now a "piece of cake". So I grew restless and wanted another "mountain to climb". What better way than to relieve or eliminate the intense misery that multiple sclerosis causes. Imagine, will you, the poor MS/whatever patient first hearing about me. They will most likely say doctors can't touch MS, what chance has this herbalist/immunologist chap. He must be some type of "nut" which of course is the exact strategy of the medical network, thus causing doubt in the mind of the would-be patient. <u>Thus an untouchable disease remains untouchable to infinity causing intolerable suffering, crippling and sometimes death.</u>

By sheer chance a person I once knew said his sister was dying of what I call fast progressive MS and doctors call it primary progressive MS where basically the poor patient can progress to a wheelchair in as little as a year or so, incontinent, suffering terribly and often dying within a few years. I thought here we go again "Gerald Green being thrown in at the deep end of the swimming bath". Almost exactly like Mrs S. of Lewes, my very first ulcerative-colitis patient who was lined up for a colostomy if I failed – only this was worse in that the MS lady was actually dying.

Some years before I was given a dirty, scruffy, little booklet which said there is a base metallic element which takes away the awful pain of rheumatoid arthritis. I am absolutely fascinated with true science and knew full well there was no way this metallic element could in itself relieve pain in this auto-immune orientated arthritis. Then the "penny dropped" and I realised this chemical, although not a pain killer, can "turn off" the immune system from, in this case, attacking the joints. Okay fine, I would use this immune ingredient for probably the very first time against MS. However, there was a problem in that the dose is only the size/weight of say three pins heads. How do you put this tiny amount of the immune ingredient into size 0 capsule (an average size capsule?) The answer was simple because I realised MS patients often suffer muscle spasms so I thought I would use a well known antispasmodic herbal powder as a carrier of the immune ingredient and what better than cramp bark powder. I then simply worked out the weight of cramp bark in a capsule, made a given number and multiplied the tiny amount of immune ingredient in a given weight of cramp bark powder so it could be mixed and correctly metered out the exact amount of milligrams a capsule.

Would it work on this terribly ill dying MS lady? I had no idea but had a gut instinct it would providing the immune-ingredients effect was not masked out by drug induced-Candida. What was the orientation and strategy behind my very first attempt at this, the very worst type of MS? Over a period of the several years I had been treating auto-immune orientated Crohn's disease and ulcerative-colitis, also studying others in the same group, I came to the conclusion, laid out clearly in the earlier part of this book, that all auto-immune orientated diseases were in fact all one and the same disease mechanism but with obvious different epicentres of immunological attack that gave these world's worst diseases their respective names. If the immune ingredient worked on rheumatoid arthritis, which it most certainly did, in a low density Candida patient, then providing the patient used the well defined anti-candida diet of no cows milk and products, yeast, gluten and above all sugar, then the immune ingredient would "turn off" immunological attack in any of this group of terrible diseases.

The fast progressive MS lady, Susan, who was close to the end of her life, incontinent and wheelchair bound for two and a half years and living a life of (if such it could be called) "living hell", was only too pleased at her brother's prompting to let me try to relieve her abject misery. She was very cooperative in carrying out the essential anti-candida diet. Within just a week she felt sensation in her limbs, her slurred speech improved and her eyesight also. I was overjoyed. Surely to God, I was not going to get this terrible disease at my first attempt like I did with my own life threatening vicious asthma and emphysema in 1976 and also Mrs S. of Lewes with her auto-immune orientated inflammatory bowel disease and by now many others with the same disease? However, Susan was fully continent within a month, taking her first steps from her wheelchair prison and her eyesight and slurred speech normalised. As far as I knew then, this had never happened before.

I was by now over the moon with enthusiasm and if anyone thinks the above is a figment of my imagination, Susan is well documented in my booklet called "Multiple Sclerosis Beaten Against All The Odds" so called because of the way the medical profession, patients' relations and yes sometimes the patients themselves were sceptical about me and thought it was impossible. One reason is that MS often attacks the brain in the "rhyme and reason" area and basically if a MS patient is so badly affected mentally, what chance then of them following the absolutely essential anti-candida diet?

 Not unnaturally often patients' relations took notice of what the doctors said to the MS patients relative to diet not being important, so preventing the very method that could win their only way out of their intense misery.

However, Susan followed the diet and went from strength to strength and eventually she walked again and had a life worth living with approximately 75% relief remission which bearing in mind how severely she was affected by primary progressive MS might well be attributed as a near miracle by many.

I was over the moon with enthusiasm to relieve more MS patients but sadly because of orthodox disregard to my treatment of MS patients and even their relations in some cases and with absolutely no help from the MS Society, I had a very depressing time due to my work not being recognised by the professional orthodox bodies.

I had all but given up hope, well documented in my MS booklet: under the heading "Four Years in the Medical Wilderness", when an Australian lady I knew, Myra Finlay, wrote an article in the mid-1990's in a Brisbane newspaper about the wonderful results I had achieved with a terribly ill MS patient against appalling odds and oppression in the UK. Now, believe me, Australia is by no means medically free but, compared to the UK's medical blackout of people in alternative medicine, it was very much freer and enlightened than the UK. When Myra's article was printed about my work in Australia and Susan's wonderful relief when dying of MS, I received six requests to be similarly relieved of their severe MS problems. To say I was overjoyed would have been the understatement of the year because here I was after four long years of medical oppression in which I could not get a single MS patient after such a wonderful result with Susan, with six Australian MS ladies all terribly affected and really wanting to improve their lot.

To cut a long story short I managed to give a very high percentage remission to five of the six MS ladies, four of which were wheelchair bound, but one would not follow the absolutely essential anti-candida diet and sadly she died. At the end of the day I am not God and if a patient, and there are rather a lot in the MS group, who will not go half way towards helping themselves with the essential dietary regime, then even I am powerless to help them if up to 100% of my medicinal effect is masked out by Candida.

Now I knew for absolute sure I had cracked MS and I wrote "Multiple Sclerosis Beaten Against All The Odds". However, things were no better in the oppressive, medically speaking, UK. So I looked further afield to New Zealand where I had taught the very successful herbalist, Mrs Pam Blowers of Whangei, my methods. She told me about a wonderful natural environmental and alternative medicine magazine called "Soil and Health" run by the then editor Mr Chris Wheeler.

Chris printed an article on my work that started in the UK and then Australia. The response was ongoing after the slow start in the UK. The New Zealanders are much more "open minded" than the often <u>orthodox "programmed" people in the UK</u>, and they would never put up with the alternative medical whitewash we get in the UK from the orthodox profession. From the wonderful publicity I had in New Zealand, a good number of MS patients applied for treatment. I now had dozens of eager Kiwi MS patients wanting treatment. Needless to say many of these patients were relieved of their misery and again I was "over the moon" with happiness.

Now naturally you would have thought the New Zealand MS Society would have been overjoyed with the MS patients getting relieved of their misery. However, their only action was to try and take Editor Chris Wheeler to court for simply having told the truth. This shows you what most disease charities can be like in my experience. Something about "killing the goose that lays the golden egg"!

Carol K

Carol K was almost blinded, eyes rolling uncontrollably as you see in blind folk, plus all of the other terrible MS symptoms mentioned in the chart below. When this lovely girl (barely able to walk) left my house with her husband, I had tears rolling down my cheeks that life could be so cruel. Yet with the combination of the essential diets and my unique MS formula that stops immunological attack on the myelin sheath in a low Candida density, Carol's awful symptoms were "cut to pieces" relative to her years of suffering with fast progressive MS "overnight". Carol's eyesight eventually returned fully over two months, first in black and white, then one colour after another to normal eyesight.

In one of her letters Carol wrote "Thank you for giving me my life back".

I have also included a second progress chart from another Carole (this one with an 'e' on the end of her name.) which follows after Carol K.

MS TREATMENT MONITORING CHART

DAY/ DATE 5th Sept. 95	0	Week 1	Week 2	Week 3	Week 4
Symptoms :					
DOUBLE VISION/OPTIC NEURITIS	S	m	SL	SL	SL
SLURRED SPEECH					
JAW UNABLE TO OPEN FULLY					
NUMB MOUTH/TONGUE/GUMS					
NUMB SCALP/FACE					
NUMB RIGHT ARM					
NUMB LEFT ARM	m	m	SL	Gone	Gone
DIZZINESS	m	SL	SL	Gone	Gone
WEAKNESS	m	SL	SL	Gone	Gone
LOSS OF BALANCE	S	m	SL	Gone	Gone
EXTREME FATIGUE	m	SL	SL	SL	Gone
HEAVINESS IN RIGHT ARM					
HEAVINESS IN LEFT ARM					
HEAVINESS IN RIGHT LEG					
HEAVINESS IN LEFT LEG	S	S	m	SL	Gone
WEAKNESS IN RIGHT HAND					
WEAKNESS IN LEFT HAND	S	m	m	SL	Gone
VERTIGO					
BLADDER INCONTINENCE					
BOWEL INCONTINENCE					
CONSTIPATION					
SPASM IN LEGS	m	SL	SL	SL	Gone
SPASMS IN ARMS	m	SL	SL	SL	Gone
LIMBS EXTREMELY COLD	S	m	SL	SL	Gone
LIMBS EXTREMELY HOT					
SENSITIVE TO CHEMICALS					
HALITOSIS (BAD BREATH)					
MIGRAINE					
EMOTIONAL PROBLEMS					
CO-ORDINATION	S	M	m	SL	Gone
SEXUAL DYSFUNCTION					
PAIN	S	SL	SL	SL	Gone

Please underline if you have ; REMITTING MS / PROGRESSIVE MS
Please indicate severity of symptoms prior to treatment in column O, for example;
S = SEVERE   M = MODERATE   SL = SLIGHT
Using this code, continue through the weeks, showing relief or lack of it and write the word GONE where relative.

Name	Carol ...
Address	
Telephone Number	
Comments;	I found the improvement very fast, which with diet & your medication I think wonderful to wonderful effect

MS TREATMENT MONITORING CHART

DAY/DATE 29/1/97	0	Week 1	Week 2	Week 3	Week 4
Symptoms					
DOUBLE VISION/OPTIC NEURITIS					
SLURRED SPEECH	m	SUCH IMPROVEMENT	GONE	GONE	
JAW UNABLE TO OPEN FULLY					
NUMB MOUTH/TONGUE/GUMS					
NUMB SCALP/FACE					
NUMB RIGHT ARM	m	IMPROVED	GONE	GONE	GONE
NUMB LEFT ARM					
DIZZINESS	m	IMPROVED	GONE	GONE	GONE
WEAKNESS	SL	IMPROVED	GONE	GONE	GONE
LOSS OF BALANCE	SL	IMPROVED	GONE	GONE	GONE
EXTREME FATIGUE	M	IMPROVED	GONE	GONE	GONE
HEAVINESS IN RIGHT ARM					
HEAVINESS IN LEFT ARM					
HEAVINESS IN RIGHT LEG	m	IMPROVED. IMPROVED	GONE	GONE	
HEAVINESS IN LEFT LEG					
WEAKNESS IN RIGHT HAND	m	IMPROVED GONE	GONE	GONE	
WEAKNESS IN LEFT HAND					
VERTIGO					
BLADDER INCONTINENCE					
BOWEL INCONTINENCE					
CONSTIPATION	SL	IMPROVED GONE	GONE	GONE	
SPASM IN LEGS	S	IMPROVED GONE	GONE	GONE	
SPASMS IN ARMS					
LIMBS EXTREMELY COLD	SL	IMPROVED GONE	GONE	GONE	
LIMBS EXTREMELY HOT					
SENSITIVE TO CHEMICALS					
HALITOSIS (BAD BREATH)					
MIGRAINE					
EMOTIONAL PROBLEMS					
CO-ORDINATION	S	GREAT IMPROVEMENT GONE	GONE	GONE	
SEXUAL DYSFUNCTION					
PAIN	S	IMPROVED GONE	GONE	GONE	

Please underline if you have ; REMITTING MS / PROGRESSIVE MS
Please indicate severity of symptoms prior to treatment in column O, for example;
S = SEVERE   M = MODERATE   SL = SLIGHT
Using this code, continue through the weeks, showing relief or lack of it and write the word GONE
where relative.

Name	CAROLE
Address	
Telephone Number	
Comments;	I FEEL GREAT, MORE HEALTHIER THAN I HAVE IN A LONG TIME, I AM ALSO FREE FROM PAIN. THANKS TO YOU. Carole

50

Carole

I don't claim I can achieve fantastic results like Carole's every time (see previous chart), in fact it's 1 in 6 with 3 in 6 massively or moderately relieved. One of the main reasons for the 50% failure rate is that although neurologists have little idea how to treat MS, most rubbish these absolutely essential diets out of sight (no money to be made in diets).

Paul M

Obviously I only have room to put in a few progress charts but feel that this one must be in there as the remarkable thing about this is that it is from a male. Generally I have found that males are not prepared to follow the strict anti-candida diet to the letter and continue to suffer as a result.

Imagine what it's like to walk again from your wheelchair "prison" and to be "clean and dry" and free of the worst of Paul's awful symptoms including 'blinding' migraines in just a few weeks.

GERALD GREEN
MEDICAL HERBALIST
& IMMUNOLOGIST
Tel. Bedall 218683 (AftEm)

MS TREATMENT MONITORING CHART

DAY/ DATE 20/3/00	0	Week 1	Week 2	Week 3	Week 4
Symptoms					
DOUBLE VISION/OPTIC NEURITIS	M	SL	SL	SL	SL
SLURRED SPEECH	SL	SL	SL	SL	SL
JAW UNABLE TO OPEN FULLY					
NUMB MOUTH/TONGUE/GUMS					
NUMB SCALP/FACE					
NUMB RIGHT ARM	SL	SL	Gone	Gone	Gone
NUMB LEFT ARM					
DIZZINESS	S	SL	SL	Gone	Gone
WEAKNESS	S	S	M	M	SL
LOSS OF BALANCE	S	S	M	M	SL
EXTREME FATIGUE	S	S	M	SL-M	SL
HEAVINESS IN RIGHT ARM					
HEAVINESS IN LEFT ARM	S	S	M	M	M
HEAVINESS IN RIGHT LEG	SL	SL	SL	SL	SL
HEAVINESS IN LEFT LEG	S	S	S	S-M	M
WEAKNESS IN RIGHT HAND	M	M	SL	SL	SL
WEAKNESS IN LEFT HAND	S	S	M	M	SL
VERTIGO					
BLADDER INCONTINENCE	M	M	SL	SL-G	Gone
BOWEL INCONTINENCE	M	M	Gone	Gone	Gone
CONSTIPATION	M	SL	Gone	Gone	Gone
SPASM IN LEGS	M	M	M	M-SL	SL
SPASMS IN ARMS					
LIMBS EXTREMELY COLD	S	S	M	M-SL	M-SL
LIMBS EXTREMELY HOT					
SENSITIVE TO CHEMICALS					
PINS AND NEEDLES	SL	SL	SL	Gone	Gone
MIGRAINE	S	M	Gone	Gone	Gone
EMOTIONAL PROBLEMS					
CO-ORDINATION	M	M	M	M-SL	SL
SEXUAL DYSFUNCTION	M	M	SL	SL-Gone	Gone
PAIN	S	M	Gone	Gone	Gone

Please underline if you have ; REMITTING MS / PROGRESSIVE MS
Please indicate severity of symptoms prior to treatment in column 0, for example;
S = SEVERE   M = MODERATE   SL = SLIGHT
Using this code, continue through the weeks, showing relief or lack of it and write the word GONE
where relative.

Name	Mr P.M
Address	
Telephone Number	
Comments;	Week1 - Happy about Head Aches Can stand quiet well

Week2 Extremely happy about not having a
Headach. Started to walk on a Zimer, altogether
feel much happier in myself

52

Systemic Lupus

Having cracked MS and relieved the abject misery this awful disease causes under orthodox treatment, I wanted to move on to even more dangerous auto-immune diseases of which systemic lupus is, in my opinion, the most dangerous of the lot. Now generally, the more dangerous and painful the auto-immune disease, the easier it is to treat, especially with female patients. The reason is simple in that if you have a bad pain in the gut, as with Crohn's and ulcerative-colitis, you want to get well as soon as possible, this being why I score heavily with remissions a plenty, especially females, who would not put a pint of beer above their life, as many males, believe it or not, will. While with systemic lupus it's so dangerous and it attacks females nine to one anyway, these patients usually follow the essential diet and as a result win their remission and quickly too.

<u>With absolutely all of the auto-immune diseases no matter what, you have to wipe out Candida in the bloodstream first,</u> so I use the finest Candida killer, namely wormwood (highly compressed) as the carrier of the immune ingredient, so that providing the patient diets correctly and removes all Candida-induced

medicinal masking, the <u>immune ingredient simply turns the immune system off from attacking whatever part of the body that particular disease attacks</u>.

Due to the mechanics involved, the only exception is inflammatory bowel disease where you need the delayed-release capsules to quickly "knock out" an immunological flare and put the patient quickly into remission. With IBD the medicine follows down the whole alimentary canal ie mouth to bowel, and the herbs are designed so as they cannot miss their target en route to switch off the attack, where as all other auto-immune diseases are more indirect).

With the above methods you can "take apart" any auto-immune disease in a very quick time indeed but you could be forgiven for thinking the medical profession condone the unnecessary suffering and death these terrible diseases cause rather then give any regard to alternative therapies/diets. All my medical orientated life they have tried to "spoke my wheel" at every opportunity, though just a couple actually helped me and they, for very obvious reasons, have to be nameless. If anyone thinks me antagonistic toward the pharma/medical network, then "by heaven" they made me like it, for how would you, my readers, feel if you could relieve to nothing or very little a host of the world's very worst diseases, yet in a supposedly "free" land you are allowed no publicity at all by any but minority news outlets. The net result of this is to let this totally unnecessary suffering and death continue.

CHAPTER 5

<u>My own salvation using my
Lung Triple Alliance Formula</u>

You have seen how I started off guided by a gifted brain and unhampered by the orthodox doctrine which would have dragged me back. Also, I had an enthusiasm for relieving abject misery to first save my own life from vicious asthma and emphysema in '76, for necessity is the mother of invention and from this everything evolved. At the time, I knew nothing about medicine but found I was dying from the vicious combination of very severe bronchial asthma and sixty per cent lung destruction called emphysema caused by the excessive internal pressures that build up in the lungs. With very severe asthma you can breathe in easily but it's very difficult to breathe out causing great pressure in the lungs that over a period of time destroys parts of the lung.

Now with my very life in jeopardy (because I knew the "score" with emphysema) I made it my job to find out as quickly as possible or I was a "dead duck". Reading sometimes fifteen hours a day and completely free of orthodox "clap trap", I quickly realised liquorice had a systemic anti-inflammatory effect on many parts of the body by inducing the renal cortex on top of each kidney to make extra cortisone which are natural steroids that "home" in on inflammation in any part of our body where it may be required. Yes I thought, I'll use liquorice as the base of any formula because, in my opinion, there can't be anything better and is well known as a lung medicine anyway. What to put with it? Well again slippery elm also has an effect on the lungs, it thins down the thick mucus that clogs the airways in asthma (sometimes called asthma plugs). In addition, I wanted a herb that would expel this mucus (called an expectorant) to clear the airways and lobelia herb seemed ideal. I put this mixture together in powder format.

At the time I could get liquorice and slippery elm in powder format but lobelia I could only get in flaked leaf form so I simply made material "tea bags" with the lobelia. So I measured in a non-stick milk saucepan a pint and a quarter of cold water and put in the lobelia "tea bag" secured with a twist fastener. This was brought to the boil, whereupon the lobelia bag was mashed to get everything out into the water (now simmer boiling I took out the bag leaving the lobelia extract in the water). Now I mixed the liquorice and slippery elm together in a plastic bag and simply added four slightly raised teaspoonfuls very carefully by gently shaking the teaspoon with one hand while stirring the simmer boiling lobelia extract water with a wooden spoon with the other (very much like making gravy). Done carefully you will get no clots, but should you do so you can always use an egg whisk to disperse them. Continue stirring while simmer boiling, count two minutes and a transformation takes place whereby the slippery elm in this mixture turns the whole lot to a thin gel. When cool this is ready for use at one sherry glassful, 3 or, when severe, 4 times a day between meals, if possible. (To get the best from lobelia it has to be heated, so cannot be encapsulated successfully.)

Within only two days I could feel the iron grip on my lungs start to release, as did the freedom in my airways. Can anyone of my readers imagine in their wildest dreams what this transformation from actually dying to getting well was like? No longer was it so difficult to breathe, indeed there were times when I doubted I would get another breath prior to this new formula – my very first which I called the lung Triple Alliance. I tried a hundred times to improve this formula and could not. So I was well again in a remarkably quick time and with the asthma gone and the emphysema it had caused unable to progress, I began to realise what the power of herbs can achieve with these wonderful results in so short a time without side-effects (when orthodox medicine failed) even though the disease left me disabled from emphysema (60% lung destruction). Even so, making up medicine and encapsulation at a later stage was not going to run me out of breath.

However, I still suffered from a seven and a half year duration duodenal ulcer, so it seemed the obvious thing to do was to use, as before, liquorice as well as slippery elm for their systemic and lubricant anti-inflammatory effect but remove the purely lung herb from my lung Triple Alliance formula, namely lobelia, which I exchanged for the very expensive golden seal, an absolutely fantastic medicine. My doctor gave me morphine to kill the awful pain of the ulcer but nothing to cure it.

My brand new gut Triple Alliance formula completely got rid of this awful gut ulcer in only four and a half weeks and in one fell swoop I had invented two similar but different formulas, one that would "take apart" any non-malignant lung disease for which orthodoxy has very limited medicines called the lung Triple Alliance that had saved my life in 1976, then the natural sequence to this was the gut Triple Alliance that could "whip" any existing gut medicine by many fold and put me on the road to tackle the two worst non-malignant gut diseases in the world Crohn's and ulcerative-colitis.

The whole idea of repeating how I came into medicine in the first place with an open mind, a good brain and make no mistake I was dying and suffering very badly indeed under orthodoxy, so necessity was the mother of invention i.e. "find the answer to your problems like quickly or you're dead." I think you will agree this is as good a learning curve as one can get and many times superior to learning in a university just to become automatic "prescription pads".   Mind you, nearly losing my life, that brought me into medicine in the first place, was not the only time the "grim reaper" tried to get me and I really hope my readers will benefit and maybe save their own lives in the future from very dangerous diseases. They don't get much more dangerous than coronary heart disease.

CHAPTER 6

<u>Coronary Heart Disease</u>

When I was born in 1930 rickets was a very common medical problem caused by poor dietary fare in the Great Depression of these times. I had rickets very badly and a lot of my time as a child was spent in a hospital gym for exercises and sitting in front of sunray machines to get vitamin D, in very short supply at the time. My mother was very doctor "programmed" and his advice to her was give your child suet puddings at least <u>three times a day</u>. Sure enough from a tiny child to when I married at thirty years I was having suet morning, noon and night which did my rickets no good at all and my vascular system even less. Sure enough in middle age I started to get coronary attacks and angina which, not unnaturally, became worse very quickly until I was getting three attacks a day entailing awful pain which felt like an "elephant sitting on my chest" for over an hour at a time.

One of the doctors I was friendly with rang me up to say Prof. X had told her I was dying from coronary disease which I confirmed saying, "I only had about two weeks left in this world." "Oh", the doctor said, "where I come from (India) they die of just about everything but rarely of coronary heart disease." I replied, "I suppose they don't live long enough because things like cholera or plague kill them first", which is my wicked sense of humour, but it upset the doctor who replied, "no, it's simply they use chilli or cayenne pepper (much the same thing) in nearly all their dishes and this acts just like 'Dino Rods' (the drain clearing people) on the people's vascular systems clearing out all the fat orientated deposits that clogs up our veins and arteries. Do you get a warning an attack is coming?" Said the doctor. "Yes", I replied, "I get a dull pain just below the rib cage, then it moves up into my chest with ever increasing pain then radiating sort of electrically up my neck and down my arms by which time I am rolling on the floor in agony." "Oh yes", says the doctor, "that's fairly classic of severe coronary disease. Now what I want you to do when the dull warning pain comes, to go out in the kitchen and put on the electric kettle, then put a teaspoonful of chilli pepper into a teacup and half fill with boiling water, stir and sip slowly."

Oh my God, I thought a teaspoonful of chilli pepper in boiling water will give me a heart attack, yet the doctor mentioned (who has to be nameless) is a very highly placed doctor indeed. Oh well, I thought, this doctor is no fool. I'll compromise with half a teaspoonful of chilli pepper in a half a teacupful of boiling water. "Sip it slowly" said the doctor and believe me it would be impossible to do it any other way as it was very very hot in both senses! By now the pain was building up into a crescendo so awful and then in a flash the intense pain was almost gone as if by the "wave of a wand".

This doctor must be a magician I thought and I was very thankful and relieved. It was one of the most fantastic experiences of my life which was shortly due to run out failing her intervention. Of course, while sipping this very hot medicine, the ingredients that dilate the coronary artery go through the back of the tongue straight into the bloodstream taking no more than twenty seconds to relieve the massive pain that was building up in my body.

Well wonderful experience it most certainly was but I would in future make sure, if possible, it never got to this stage by encapsulating the chilli pepper and taking one capsule 3 times a day.

Please follow important instructions to prevent problems

Swallow capsule with water having a meal on the table ready to eat and in this way prevent the only side-effect possible, namely getting a chilli capsule stuck in the gullet which, I assure you, is not an experience anyone would want! You see, once swallowed into the stomach it's totally safe from causing discomfort because in the actual stomach there is hydrochloric acid which turns our chewed up food into a pre-digestive soup called chyme. To prevent this acid burning into our stomach's flesh there is a thick covering of mucus which protects us as well from the hot capsules naturally. By the time the capsules contents have been in the stomach three hours the intense heat (which does not burn as say a stove does) will be mellowed and no unwanted side-effects will take place.

Well I did exactly as above and basically the coronary attacks became less severe and wider apart until they went for, hopefully ever, some nine years ago. So you see by this very simple method you can get rid of possibly the most dangerous disease in the world relative to the vast numbers of people it kills or like me tortured with awful pain. I have a high IQ relative to my German scientist grandfather Prof. Fritz Haber 1868-1934 but during my terrible suffering time with coronary heart disease my brain "fogged" up and I was very forgetful. All that saturated fat had "loused up" my whole vascular system (c/o my rickets days) and basically, whatever, does not get blood and oxygen, deteriorates including the power of my brain. However when the chilli pepper had "Dino Rodded" out my whole vascular system, not only was my coronary disease gone, but I had a brain like a computer again!

There is a book called "Left for Dead" by Dick Quinn ISBN 0963283901 amazon.com £10 which is the true story of Dick whose mother died in her late twenties of a stroke and his dad died of a coronary at the age of thirty five. Now obviously genetically Dick did not stand a "dogs chance" of a long life and at thirty five he too got coronary disease, had open heart surgery but the operation was not successful. He was told about a wonderful old chap by the name of Dr. Christopher who told Dick about the wonderful powers of chilli pepper clearing out the whole vascular system but although the cardiac surgeon had done a rather poor operation on Dick he was still rather doctor "programmed" and found chilli pepper doing so much to get rid of fat deposits in the vascular system and completely relieving coronary disease rather hard to take in. (So did I initially).

Whatever, two months went by and Dick started to go blind because his optic nerve was not getting enough blood and oxygen. Realising at last old Dr. Christopher was right, Dick put all the capsules his doctor was giving him on the table, emptied out the contents which went down the toilet as they were doing no good at all. He then filled up the now empty capsules with red chilli pepper and took one 3 times a day.

Very soon, Dick's health improved in an unbelievable way as his vascular system was cleared out and blood and oxygen could again get to where it was needed. He eventually became as fit as almost anyone, completely losing his coronary disease. His eyesight, brain and just about everything improved beyond Dick's wildest dreams, <u>exactly like my own experience</u>. I think all my readers will agree the above facts re possibly the most dangerous disease in the world is well worth knowing. Perhaps by now you can see how my knowledge of medicine was evolving fast, with sometimes me being the actual patient to bring about this really true research.

<u>High Blood Pressure</u>

Not long after this experience the grim reaper had another go at me through a genetic problem handed down from my mother, namely malignant hypertension or if you like "right off the normal scale" of high blood pressure. You don't need to be told again this is a very very dangerous disease like above that causes many deaths and the maiming of patients after they have had strokes caused by the brain being flooded by blood when the high blood pressure blows out a capillary. My mother often complained in her last years of a left-side headache. Eventually she had a stroke which turned my mother into a vegetative state for five days and she finally died of a cerebral haemorrhage explained above. Then, as I reached her age, (bearing in mind I had never had a headache in my life) sure enough I started to get the same left-side headaches my mother complained about.

Knowing high blood pressure had killed my mother, I at once took my blood pressure and "lo and behold" it was "right off the scale" at systolic 220, while the diastolic pressure was 128 (for my age early '70s at the time a good BP would be systolic 120 with diastolic 80.) I told my doctor about my "off the scale" high blood pressure and he gave me some medication for it which was the strongest he had. All I can say is the truth in that when blood pressure is as high as mine was, a medicine or medicines as there were several which only takes off twenty points off of the mercury scale – or if you like reduced my systolic from 220 to 200 and my diastolic from 128 to 115 it still left me in stroke territory.

I sat down in a chair to sum up the situation, which at the time, looked dire indeed. You see although by now very skilled in most of the world's worst diseases, I have to admit I knew very little about "off the mercury scale" high blood pressure. I looked up Blacks Medical Dictionary as it says the majority of causes of high blood pressure are vague though kidney disease and ingesting too much salt are contributory factors. As these latter problems were not relevant this was not much help at all. So I sat in my chair rather despondent thinking I could "go the same way" as my poor mother.

Then a very strange thing happened (and this is not the only case). I went to read a herbal book and it fell on the floor open. I picked it up and the very first thing I read on the open pages was under the unwanted side-effects of the herb, barberry – "can cause a hazardous drop in blood pressure". My God I thought if I had a hazardous drop in my blood pressure it might put me right, as it was 210 systolic and 120 diastolic on the mercury scale of my wrist monitor machine. I also had the left-side headache which is why I was so despondent. So I rushed upstairs where I keep my herbal powders, getting a bag of barberry powder which I use for several problems but I knew nothing of its fantastic power to reduce blood pressure if my book was correct? I took a heaped teaspoonful of barberry powder mixed in water (never put any powder in your mouth dry, because if you were to cough, sneeze or do some other involuntary action it could pull the dry power in your lungs causing you to cough and splutter) about two grams and although rather bitter was, I thought, worth the research.

Within only ten minutes my "left-side headache" had almost gone as the very high blood pressure was relieved. When the medicine is taken in water like this, it obviously goes under the tongue where it can be absorbed into the bloodstream very quickly indeed and that's why it worked so quickly on my blood pressure inducing headache. Then overjoyed at the result so far, at about an hour I took my blood pressure on my wrist monitor and it was, believe it or not, systolic 120 and diastolic 80 normal for my age of 76. Yes the blood pressure had dropped by a remarkable 90° systolic and 40° diastolic in an hour <u>which is more by far than any orthodox medicine could achieve.</u>

I want my readers to think about the thousands of stroke victims and deaths caused by this devilish disease that could so easily be corrected and quickly by this wonderful herb. Also, I think of my poor mother whose stroke reduced this intelligent woman into a vegetative state for five days before it killed her. Often these poor souls continue after a stroke for years in this vegetative state which is horrible for the patient, their relations and the nursing staff that look after them and, as you can see, it's not necessary. I've told doctors about what I do, and I know they are amazed, but they have to "dance the puppet strings the pharmaceuticals pull", if you follow my drift and are non-committal.

CHAPTER 7

Cancer

Now in my fairly long life time I suppose I knew approx. some thirty people with cancer and although most had chemotherapy or radiotherapy, almost all died within a few months/years, so not unnaturally I thought cancer must be very difficult and because I was so busy with my auto-immune disease patients I thought it better to leave it well alone. This was until my own brother, Fred, got prostate cancer.

Fred (who was four years older than me) and I never got on even when we were kids. However, I did not want him to die from a disease as horrible as cancer, and I offered my services. He replied, "what do you know about cancer?" I replied, "I have taken apart many of the world's very worst diseases and I am absolutely certain I know its mechanism and that's exactly as in my auto-immune diseases, Candida is an absolute key player." "No way", he said, "the doctors will cure me."

Throughout this book I have said that often male patients tend to be doctor "programmed" (as was my brother Fred) and will rarely contribute toward their own salvation with the anti-candida diet or anything else, especially if it entails they can't have a pint of beer (even if their life was at stake). However, just over a year after diagnosis of prostate cancer he had to go to Guys Hospital to have a lung removed which shows how "cured" he was. Soon after he took on that sallow yellow look which shows the cancer now involves the liver. Yet Fred would not let me help him saying to me: "You have not been to Oxford or Cambridge University like the doctors." I replied, "if I had been to the above universities I would have been prescribing exactly what the doctors have given you – which, shall we say, has not been successful." That shut him up for a while and I believe at least got him thinking about what I had told him about getting nearly all my diseases at my first attempt, including my own killer diseases.

Eventually, the cancer spread all over poor Fred and was now in his bones. Now as my readers may or may not know, bone cancer secondaries differ from any other cancer in that it hurts like hell (like being pulled apart in the rack). Also, when, as in this case, the primary prostate cancer reaches the bones, the patient may not have long to go i.e. five days to several weeks at the outside. Now at this late stage Fred rang me up and said, "come over and do your worst." Yes he was like that and the one and only reason he called for my help was he was in agony and I was his only chance. So once again "I was thrown in at the deep end of the pool" but while that may well have frightened some people – for me it was a challenge and as always I was in to win, come what may. So I gave him what I call the "cancer kit" and the dietary chart saying to him, as I do all my patients, "the all important diet is equally as important as the medication otherwise nothing will work as in my other entire world's worst diseases." "Okay" Fred replied, "this awful pain will keep me on course of your regime." For once I realised the poor chap was telling the truth for no way would he ever let me treat him, had he not been in absolute agony and having only a very short time left.

Now at least I was in with a chance, most would have said a "dogs chance", remembering this was my first attempt ever at tumour cancer, though I had been successful with awful skin cancers some ten years prior. Well Fred must have "done the dietary regime to the letter" because in only one week all of his extreme pain from his bone cancer secondaries was gone. Yes I was "over the moon" yet again and even Fred now out of his awful pain was brimming with enthusiasm. Oh it was absolutely brilliant and this gave me possibly the greatest buzz ever.

Now if you think that was a remarkable result, in only Fred's second week of treatment, he lost his ghastly sallow, yellow pallor which proved to me his liver secondaries were dying instead of him. On his third week's treatment his full colour had come back and most of his former extreme weakness had gone.

Some seven months before he became so very ill he and my sister-in-law had booked a Mediterranean cruise and now there was a real chance that they might well go on it so they rang up the firm to say they were going on the cruise. So it was all set up and at the end of the one month's treatment, with no exaggeration at all, Fred was in easily 85% relief remission and when he came back from the cruise he was in 100% relief remission which to me was the proverbial "icing on the cake". Naturally I told him to be careful with his diet on the ship and he did because the memory of all that awful pain was fresh in his mind. I told him to keep to the diet and medication to infinity as it did not cost him a lot, especially realising his former terrible situation.

However, after two and a quarter years in 100% relief remission Fred phoned me to say "no-one could say I have cancer now. I am cured and want to pack up the diet and medication" (as though to spite me and after everything I had told him to the contrary). Well it was as I had thought the memory of that awful pain was fading fast and being basically weak, like most males, went back to ingesting all the wrong foods and drinks and combined with packing up his wormwood medication caused the former hostile to cancer bodily environment to change to one of "milk and honey" to cancer cells (everyone has them) and you don't need telling that once his bodily environment changed, back came the cancers again and he died within six months, a completely unnecessary waste of life.

My brother was my very first tumour cancer case and overall I was more than pleased with the initial result, even if he did "louse" it all up and undo a minor miracle by ignoring my advice.

<u>Daniel my Dog</u>

My second cancer case came soon after my brother first came to me for treatment when my beloved little Yorkshire Terrier, Daniel, started drinking excessively. I immediately suspected a kidney problem. Now Daniel's fur was long rather like a "mop" as Yorkies have, hiding a lump. However, the vet's fingers found it when I went to see him. The vet told me to feel the lump half the size of a hen's egg which in a little Yorkie of only four and a half pounds was large. "I'm afraid your dog has a kidney tumour and it's too far advanced for treatment and I would advise to put him to sleep."

I worshipped the ground Daniel stood on and the vet's voice stuck into my heart with shock. "No you 'bxxxdy' won't" I replied. "I've just saved my brother's life with herbs and if it works with humans it's going to work with animals." It was just a case of scaling down the dose of wormwood capsules that suited my seventeen stone brother to a four and a half pound Yorkshire Terrier. Luckily I had some tiny empty capsules I use on little children doctors could do nothing with. So I filled these little capsules and used a dose of one small capsule mixed in dog food twice a day and awaited results. It had to be seen to be believed because Daniel's large tumour halved in size in only three and a half days, while by a week it was gone completely! Many times people/medics have said to me "how on earth could it have worked so quickly?" My reply, was "humans often cheat on the essential anti-candida diet, but my little dog could not and everyone was on strict instruction not to give Daniel doggie chocolate drops, mints etc. because that would have been the sugar "kiss of death" that would have masked out all or most medicinal effects.

There was much to be learned from Daniel's case that irrespective of how severe the cancer is, if the diet can be, as in his case, entirely controlled, then I would win remission in most cases and I am obviously talking about my terminal cancer cases well beyond any doctor or in Daniel's case vet. Well Daniel was thirteen when he had that awful kidney cancer and I kept up his wormwood medication and diet for the rest of his life and he lived on in 100% relief remission. He finally passed away aged seventeen and a half years peacefully in his sleep which is approx. one hundred and ten in our years which I think speaks for itself of what can be done in a controlled case! Sadly, I cannot obviously control human patients in the same way as with that wonderful little dog so I could win remission most times.

I want you to remember many orthodox drugs, especially the ones most used for serious diseases, kill off the good bowel bugs that keep Candida in control it being its food source. This is exactly why drugs for the world's very worst diseases eventually sends them out of control because Candida in its parasitic fungal format masks out some or all the medicinal effects causing them to be the world's very worst diseases as proof absolute of what I'm saying. Sometime have a think about the many diseases there are and how many medicines actually cure a problem and you will find you can quickly count the few there are.

Charlie

I do just want to mention again the importance of the strict anti-Candida diet and include here the sad story of a beautiful little girl called Charlotte (Charlie - aged 4).

Long before I had worked out the mechanisms of cancer (and my brother's case) a father who had heard about my reputation with deadly diseases asked me to help his little daughter Charlie and travelled some way to come and see me. I was honest and said I had not treated cancer, let alone a deadly brain tumour like she had called gilo blastoma, where life expectancy can be very short.

My older readers may remember the French singer Maurice Chevalier singing "Thank heavens for little girls" – also being "sugar and spice and all things nice". Well Charlie was all of those things and more bless her and there was no way she was going to die without a fight – but where was I going to start? Even in those earlier days, I knew Candida was the absolute key player in all of the World's very worst diseases so it would obviously follow it would be heavily implicated in cancer also.

I explained to her dad that he would have to be strong in discipline because of what is called cancer's sweet tooth which most in alternative medicine know about. What they do not all know about and almost no-one in orthodoxy, is that the real reason for very ill patients craving sugar and products, is that it's Candida that causes the problem by ingesting the patient's own blood sugar which, as explained earlier, it converts into alcohol that fuels the cancer tumours. In so doing and with so much alcohol in the blood stream, the patient's body becomes a slave to this drug and they become pseudo alcoholics who crave not alcohol but sugar which of course massively increases Candida's population within the patient. This in turn parasitizes ever more blood sugar (causing extreme fatigue) and produces ever increasing amounts of alcohol giving the body its 'fix' in drug terminology.

Subtle I think is the word and it's the very real reason some cancers race through patients, including my lovely little Charlie up 'til now. Chemo had been used on her but was documented as not being successful. However, on my anti-Candida diet alone, she had three years in remission. Then I heard her dad was persuaded to let her have chemo again by the Oncologist and Charlie sadly died.

During the time Charlie came to see me she begged her dad to let her take my little Yorkshire Terrier Daniel home (like a toy). This was of course the dog Daniel mentioned earlier who was my second cancer patient and who won his remission in only one week in a case too far gone for a vet.

CHAPTER 8

My Success with a Doctor!

Continuing on the cancer theme there is a nameless doctor whose life I saved from the multiple-allergy syndrome (caused by the Candida orientated leaky-gut syndrome) who came to hear of my success with "terminal" cancer and he phoned me to say, like any GP, he had loads of dying cancer patients, could I help. "You 'bet your boots' I can" I replied, for this you see was exactly what I wanted, namely lots of terminal patients with many different cancers to see if my medicines and dietary regime were equally effective against all cancers. So I sent off several of what I call my "cancer kits" to the doctor.

The very first patient was a lady in her early seventies who looked pregnant except it was caused by a huge bowel cancer in about as terminal case as one can get even for me. The doctor gave her my medication and instruction chart which left no one in doubt about the importance of the vital diet without which nothing could be achieved. About two weeks later while driving and doing his rounds the doctor thought he would call on Mrs X fully expecting for her to have either passed away or a Macmillan nurse to answer the door bell.

Well you can imagine the doctor's surprise when it was Mrs X herself answering the door! He was even more surprised to see her massive stomach was flattened and that she had colour in her cheeks. "Oh doctor I feel so much better", she said to my amazed doctor friend. He said, "do you mind if I come in and examine you?" "Of course", she replied and all the doctor could find was a lot of sagging, loose stomach flesh rather like a women who had just had a baby, but obviously not in her case. To cut a long story short the lady made progress equally as fast as did my brother and was soon in remission from her former death bed of by now only a month's time and thus it went on with several of the doctors "terminal" cancer patients. Of course I could not save everyone, nor could I be a fly on the wall seeing if they carried out the dietary regime correctly.

Imagine, if your doctor told you the essential diet was rubbish and naturally you are very very ill indeed like all my patients, what would you think and do? Probably you would not diet and therefore ultimately be responsible for your own demise. My experience with my doctor friend's many patients with as many different cancers I saved, was that every single one was dying with only a few days/weeks to go.

Then very unexpectedly a problem arose with the pharma/medical network. I, and I doubt anyone else could have imagined except those who know how mercenary this network really is. There were a number of different oncologists relative to the above doctor friend and my mutual cancer patients, often when seeing a terribly ill patient who has only a few weeks left give a humouring goodbye saying they will see them again in "two months time". Now there's nothing wrong with this "white lie" as anything at all that can raise the patient's spirits can't be bad. However, when these dying patients became suddenly well naturally many were amazed. This was especially so when oncologists saw their patients turn up for an appointment they thought would be impossible for them and, if anything, were fitter than their oncologist!

Now this should not happen in real every day life, especially as these different oncologists rang one another up on the phone re their amazing facts of formerly dying patients suddenly getting totally well. They knew there must be a common factor or denominator associated with all these cases and of course this was my GP friend. Far from being praised for helping save some of his dying cancer patients way-way beyond the skills of any orthodox treatment anywhere, he was lucky not to have got "struck off" the medical register. He was severely reprimanded by the all powerful medical network for being associated with me.

I went on to treat a young lady who had breast cancer, first treated several years prior at the Royal Marsden Hospital who had told her she was "cured". Sadly, when the orthodox profession talks about cures their claim is limited, often meaning anything from eighteen months to a few years before it comes back again. Don't you, my readers, think it far more honest and fairer to call the relief given <u>remission?</u>

However, when this lady was referred to me by word of mouth through another lady I had also saved from breast cancer, she was absolutely riddled with multiple secondary cancers including liver and bone cancers affecting the skull, shoulder blades, spine, chest, ribs, femur and knee caps. She was told if she had further chemotherapy etc. it might prolong her life for a year or two – <u>if it worked</u> re what little time she had left.

Well Mrs N, as I'll call her, started her treatment with me and at five months she had to go for a check up at the Royal Marsden Hospital. By now all of her terrible symptoms were gone so she knew it would be a good result. Her oncologist confirmed there was a significant reduction in her multiple secondary cancers all over her body and the really awful pain caused by her many bone cancers were long gone. I should explain bone cancer secondaries differ from most in that they "hurt like hell". So I use them where relevant as an <u>indicator as to how my medicines and dietary regime are working</u>.

A very good sign is that all this associated excruciating bone cancer pain has gone in only one week, like with my brother and many others. It also tells me if the patient is carrying out the essential diet correctly because without it there would be no beneficial result and most doctors, as said, rubbish this absolutely vital anti-candida diet showing how misguided they are. Well Mrs N left the RM Hospital full of the joys of life bless her re. her miraculous result beyond her wildest dreams. (Although told not to say this by the consultant, it's the God's truth so I'll say it and it was this quote – "I don't know who's treating you but whoever it is stick with him)."

It only goes to show you even amongst the most arrogant intransigent professions there are a few good ones - who says I've never a good word to say about doctors, well there's one! Mrs N. went to the Royal Marsden Hospital on the 12-12-02 for a check up and was told by her oncologist she was clear of her primary breast and multiple secondary cancers. I was overjoyed with the news of her very fast recovery from as "terminal" as you will get a mass of cancers like with Mrs N.

Just prior to this wonderful case I was asked to help a terribly ill cancer patient, actually the editor of the Soil and Health Magazine, Chris Wheeler's sister, (who gave me the wonderful publicity in New Zealand relative to multiple sclerosis mentioned earlier in this book). Well you will remember that time after time I get seemingly impossible cancer cases with not many days/weeks to get a result in. Here we go again when Chris Wheeler rang me up from New Zealand to say his sister was desperately ill in hospital in Australia with cancer of the uterus with again loads of secondaries and not expected to live more than two weeks remembering even if, as I did, send the medication to Australia by airmail it would take at least a week to nine days leaving me with approx. six days of life left to save her.

So I rang them to start the diet immediately and her relations smuggled the necessary food into the hospital. Yes, I thought they may well get away with smuggling in food into hospital to start Nora on the diet but no way will the medics allow my encapsulated wormwood and astragalus to be used on her. So I rang her husband saying that as everyone including the medics knew Nora was dying, tell her to ask the medics to be allowed to go home to die, then we would have the freedom to do what I knew to be correct, and not to be harassed by medics who would not have a clue as how to save a cancer patient way way beyond any orthodox treatment in this world. Poor Nora by now was so very weak she could only use a wheelchair and had to have assistance to shower, toilet etc. etc.

Once at home I knew we were in with a chance of saving Nora because her brother, Chris Wheeler, had told her "Gerald can tackle just about anything really lethal and absolutely loves the challenge involved". As Nora was so emaciated, initially she could only take very small meals often. Yet in only three weeks from being at "deaths door" she could walk again climbing eight stairs to the dining room for her now near normal size meals. She was able to wash and shower, make her own bed and even help dry the dishes!

Every day from the start of my treatment Nora grew stronger and in the words of her husband and relations her recovery was amazing and had to be seen to be believed. By a month, Nora was eating full meals, her complexion had returned to normal rosy colour from that horrible yellowish grey it had been, indeed in so little time she was almost exactly like other patients of mine you've read about. Nora went back to hospital for a check up and her doctor almost "fell out of his chair" with utter amazement (without asking how or why this new miracle had happened).

Doctors, because of the restraints of their professions, are very like politicians and sadly refused to acknowledge this 'miracle'. Yet I have conferred with the world's top doctors who have seen the proof absolute of what I have achieved against terrible odds. However, the harder they attacked me, the harder I fought and I know full well I would never have achieved so much but for what I felt were their antagonistic actions. Eventually Nora went back to the Australian countryside with friends full of the joys of life.

See progress chart from Nora and letter from her sister-in-law Margaret

Large Tumour in uterus with secondaries attached to bowel and bladder.
Secondaries remaining after hysterectomy.

Suggested Medical Treatment
Chemotherapy with all its side effects, but not expected to be
successful.
Hormone treatment which MAY slow down the growth of the tumour.
Very strong pain killers which make her too "dopey" to manage her life –
again with side effects but NO CURE.

UNDER THEIR DOCTOR

CANDIDA Treatment Monitoring Chart

Date Started Treatment: 1 - 3 - 2001   TREATMENT WITH GERALD GREEN

Wk 0	Symptoms	Wk 2	Wk 4	Wk 6	Wk 8	Wk 10
S	NAUSEA	GONE				
S	CONSTIPATION	GONE				
S	DIARRHOEA	M	GONE			
S	LACK OF APPETITE	SL	GONE			
S	PHYSICAL DEBILITY	S	M	GONE		
S	EXTREME ANXIETY	S	M	SL	GONE	
S	PAIN	S	M	SL	GONE	

What is your main illness?   CANCER

Please indicate the severity of the symptons prior to treatment in Column "0" above, in the following manner:

S = SEVERE; M = MODERATE; SL = SLIGHT

Using this simple code, continuing through the weeks, showing relief or lack of it and write the word "GONE" where relative

Name: NORA	
Address:	
Telephone No: AUSTRALIA	

Comments: This has been an astonishing result to go
from death's door to good health in such a short
time, with no bad side effects, is no less than
miraculous. Medical profession – PLEASE TAKE NOTE.

PTO

89

NORA PETERS   Progress Report

Address

ᵢ Australia   3106

Date of birth 11-10-1929

Nora suffered from a massive tumour in the uterus.

She underwent a radical hysterectomy on February 14th 2001 The main part of the tumour was removed but the doctors said that the tumour had been attached to the bladder and the bowel   and they had not got all of it. She suffered from constipation alternating with diarrhoea . She was unable to eat as she was constantly nauseous. She could walk only with the aid of a wheeled walking trolley and then only for a few yards.

The doctors recommended chemotherapy

Nora heard of the wonderful results Gerald Green had been achieving with the use of wormwood and an anti candida diet

As Nora was in hospital and very ill at that time she asked her brother, Bryan to contact Gerald.

We were all very impressed and excited so Nora decided to embark on this treatment

She informed the doctors that she did not want to have chemotherapy. They accepted this without pressure One of the doctors involved with her,later told me that the reason for the lack of pressure was because they didn't believe it   (chemotherapy) would do any good, but they had to offer it !

She commenced the diet immediately

(Food had to be smuggled into the hospital , as naturally the food there was mainly unsuitable)

She commenced taking the wormwood capsules on 1st March 2001.

She was released from hospital on the 8th March 2001 It was necessary to take her out to the car in a wheelchair.

She was unable to walk unaided , to shower herself ,or go unaided to the toilet.

At first she was able to eat only very small meals. So she had lots of them. Essentially she grazed –

Always within the boundaries of the diet., exactly as instructed by Gerald. And of course she was taking the wormwood as instructed

The progress was amazing Each day she became stronger, each day she was able to eat more., As instructed ,by Gerald she supplemented her diet with Echinacea, and Astragalus,

She was concerned about the number of bowel motions she was having – about six per day but as they were normal motions, Gerald assured her that this was the body's way of dealing with eliminating the toxins from the cancer

Three weeks after the commencement of the full treatment Nora was able to climb the eight stairs to come up to the dining room for her meals. She was showering herself, washing her hair ,making her own bed and even helping dry the dishes. Wonderful progress !

Her appetite had increased to the stage that she was eating as much as her brother Bryan, who is a very hearty eater !

Her complexion had by then lost that grey pallor and returned to her normal quite rosy colour.

Bowel motions had reduced to four per day.

Her weight had stabilized . She had not actually gained weight at that stage but then the anti-candida diet is hardly a "fat-gaining diet" !

She then returned to live in the country with friends. She still rigidly maintained the diet.

She has continued to gain strength and energy .

By the time she returned to the hospital's out-patient clinic in April for her post operative check she was walking **two kilometres** per day

The doctor was astounded at her progress (without asking how or why)

It has been a most remarkable experience to witness Nora's recovery

We are all very mindful of Gerald's warning that we should regard this as Remission.

Nora is determined to maintain this unique treatment for the rest of her life.

It is impossible to thank Gerald Green adequately for his quite remarkable work in this field and for his accessibility and dedication. We hope many , many others have the same success and that eventually this treatment receives the mainstream acceptance it deserves.

Margaret Wheeler

I am also including another letter and progress chart from a young lady, Nicci, who I treated with primary breast cancer with multiple secondaries all over her body plus extensive bone cancer.

Address:

Telephone:

Date of birth: 9 March 1969

At the age of 27, I was diagnosed with breast cancer. I underwent a right side lumpectomy, followed by six months of chemotherapy and 5 weeks of radiotherapy. After this period, I was told I was in remission.

I had six years free from the disease but in August 2001, I started to feel unwell. I rang the hospital saying I was having pains in various places but they said to just keep my appointment in September and they would see me then. This was subsequently cancelled until the day after Boxing Day. By this time, the cancer had spread to a large number of areas.

My diagnosis was secondary bone cancer re primary. I had tumours on my skull, shoulder blades, spine, chest, ribs, hips, femurs and knee caps. There was also a lesion showing in my liver but having had two scans, no one department would say whether it was cancer or not as they could not decide.

Given my diagnosis, I was told by a doctor at the Royal Marsden Hospital in London, a specialist oncologist hospital, that the best I could expect to have left was two years if the treatment they gave me was to work and prolong my time left.

I was lucky enough to be given Gerald's number by a lady who had also had breast cancer. I went to visit Gerald and he began to explain to me all about diet and how this affects us.

I immediately commenced the diet and began taking the wormwood capsules.

After five months of following this regime, I went for some more scans. When I went to visit the doctor at the Royal Marsden for my results it was the same doctor who had said I could only hope for two years. She went onto say that the scans had shown a significant reduction in all tumour sites and some by more than over 50%. I knew that the results would be good because, since starting the diet and wormwood, I have felt so much better. The extreme boney pain is now no longer existent and all other symptoms are gone.

I realise that I must maintain this way of eating for the rest of my life but I feel it is a small price to pay in order to have a life. Having a daughter of only 7 years old, I do not feel she should be left without her mummy just for the sake of say, a piece of chocolate. I really do not miss my old ways of eating and now thoroughly enjoy my food.

If at any time you should wish to contact me to talk to me in order that I can reconfirm my results, I would be more than happy for you to do so.

Gerald is passionately committed to his work and for someone of his age this is not just a hobby or experiment. He knows it works, I am proof of that and it would only be for the good of every cancer patient if Gerald's treatments were allowed to be used in hospitals who treat cancer patients.

NICCI

GG – Nicci was declared clear of all of her primary breast and multiple secondary cancers by the Royal Marsden Hospital on the 12-12-02. Because Nicci is a young woman and her hormones are high, it makes for the most aggressive cancers there are. However, middle aged and elderly patients have low hormones therefore the cancers are often destroyed in half the time of Nicci's.

This is what gives me a buzz. Indeed to save lives like this is becoming ever more common and to me is like an addictive drug.

93

Leukaemia

While I had been very successful with normal tumour cancer in its 'terminal' format, I desperately wanted to have a go at leukaemia, especially a deadly type I had heard about called acute myeloid leukaemia which 'takes no prisoners'.

A lady read about me on the internet relative to my work with cancer. She explained that her husband Roly was dying in hospital of acute myeloid leukaemia. OK I thought, that was exactly the scenario I might be able to help with because he was dying in hospital and feeling naturally terrible and frightened, so just maybe (being a male) he would not 'belly-ache' about the essential diet.

His wife told him about me and my reputation with terrible diseases and he agreed to let me try to get him in remission but, as is the norm, time was fast running out for Roly. I used my usual strategy, suggesting him being allowed to die with dignity at home because once out of hospital we might well be able to help him.

At exactly the same time I offered to help Roly, a strange coincidence happened in that first in the magazine 'The New Scientist' and a week later the Daily Mail, there were two articles about a herb feverfew which my readers may know is a brilliant migraine herb. However the article was about a powerful extract of feverfew which could kill leukaemia cells in a most exciting and almost unbelievable way.

As some may know, stem cells are able to replicate themselves into almost anything the body may require. They also create lymphocytes which, as I have mentioned, are a valuable part of our immune system and are in reality immunological 'soldiers' without which we could not exist because of the vital protection they provide.

Black's medical dictionary states "the cause of leukaemia is not known", but I read in the two articles mentioned above that sometimes stem cells have their DNA altered causing them to over-produce the immunological soldiers like lymphocytes en-masse and it is that massive over production that are called leukaemia cells.

We all hear about heat seeking missiles that cannot miss their target, well here we can see nature trying to emulate that because the powerful feverfew extract can seemingly differentiate between the rogue stem cells (pro-creating leukaemia cells) and the normal stem cells that have not had their DNA altered that produce, in this case, normal essential lymphocytes. Therefore, as always, I go "for the throat" of the enemy and gave the patient the powerful feverfew extract, plus the essential diet and wormwood to kill Candida and await events.

Roly, who had been sent home to die, was suddenly running about like the proverbial 'blue arse fly'! with again a remarkable recovery, with the immunological battle being won quickly too, at my very first attempt at leukaemia.

Readers may well say if the rogue stem cells over-produce lymphocytes en masse all to the good with these millions of extra immunological soldiers. This is not so and it is best to compare say an apple tree over-producing (and they can) a thousand tiny apples the size of marbles that are no good to anyone. It's similar with these tiny useless lymphocytes which cannot do their job of killing the enemy and so the body breaks down as the immune system is 'clapped out'.

I told Norman, a mutual friend of Pam Blowers in New Zealand, about my success with leukaemia and he tried out exactly what I did on a high ranking clergyman who was dying, just the same as Roly. He got the same result as me, proving it was not just a "flash in the pan".

Indeed, doctors and consultants in New Zealand had never seen anything like it before – but in future they now most likely will!

The orthodox medics would say how could you form a result like that without a double-blind trial? The answer is <u>"I do it all the time"</u> because my dying and very seriously ill patients have only days or weeks at the outside to live and they can't wait umpteen years for trials to be carried out. The results of which are often questionable as has recently been proved with an anti-depressant drug which was shown to be no better than the placebo or say sugar pills and any result was purely the faith the patient had in their doctor.

Often orthodox medical-orientated journalists in many newspapers accuse us of only being able to create a placebo effect. Well, all I can say, is just you try and "placebo" a wheelchair bound MS patient suffering terribly, back to not only being able to walk again, but going on to marry, have children and eventually hold down a good job – an impossibility under orthodox medicine. Then and then only can you say you have medicines and methods that really do work like no other!

CHAPTER 9

<u>Skin Cancers</u>

Although this section on cancer is about what I've achieved in the majority of main line cancers, I've made no mention of skin cancers which I have been treating successfully for over twenty years with a lotion made from the stepped up extract of the greater celandine herb.

<u>This does not need any of the dietary requirements as with main line cancers</u> and is treatable just with a celandine lotion treatment.

In some parts of the country it's called the wart plant because its bright orange juice destroys warts better than anything I know. Within hours of seeing how successful it was on a young school boy who's hands were covered in warts (he was too embarrassed to go to school), I thought, could this work on skin cancer?

<u>Mr Brewster</u>

At about this time, my wife and I went on an outing and we were sitting next to an elderly gentleman at our hotel table. His hands and face were covered in horrible wart like growths to almost cauliflower proportions. I felt so sorry for him, especially when he said "if you find me too embarrassing, I'll go to another table". I'm sure by now you can be thinking what I replied! I said "you stay where you are because I want to know what your problem is and see if I can do something about it". (It would be no exaggeration to say this poor old chap made Frankenstein look pretty.) He replied that he had a type of skin cancer called squamous cell carcinoma.

I asked what treatment his specialist gave him. When the growths became too large they cut them out leaving, as was clear to see, a crater nearly down to his skull bone that did nothing to enhance this poor man's looks. <u>By now I was boiling in anger that this sort of thing could happen in our day and age to such a nice old gent</u> called Mr Brewster.

Please remember I had never treated any sort of cancer twenty years ago but I was so horrified with what I saw, I was going to crack this loathsome disease or 'die in the attempt'. As good as the greater celandine is I did not think it would be powerful enough to rid Mr Brewster's multiple afflictions so the only thing to do was to step up the celandine's strength in a similar way to how some wines are stepped up to become fortified wines. I used surgical spirit to get the initial extract from one lot of celandine herb and when that was done, put another lot of this herb in the resultant extract to double, treble and finally four fold the strength of the celandine until it was dark brown in colour - almost black.

I tested it out on myself first to check for side effects and apart from stains which washed off eventually, there were none. I then phoned up Mr Brewster to see if he would let me treat him and not surprisingly he was only too pleased someone cared enough to do this.

I used an artist's paintbrush once a day to cover the hundreds of growths that mainly affected the whole head and hands. After only two weeks, the smaller of the growths were falling off, roots and all, so it was obvious that the celandine lotion was chemically opposed to the cancer and was passing through the skin (osmosis) into the roots of the cancer.

I was absolutely delighted as was Mr Brewster! However, Teutonic to a fault for those that know me, everything has to be done quickly, efficiently and no matter what I do, am never satisfied until I reach perfection and next time I did. I reasoned that when I painted the celandine lotion on Mr Brewster's multiple facial head and hand cancers, it soon dried on them and as such made its passage through the cancer and skin to get at and destroy the roots via osmosis less efficient than if it was kept wet or damp when it would work continuously.

I explained to Mr Brewster my strategy to speed things up a bit by painting his cancers as before but while still wet, covered them with plastic film and taped them in place. Obviously it sweated under the plastic and being permanently damp, worked 24 hours a day so that by after only one month's treatment, Mr Brewster was 100% clear of all of his multiple facial, head and hand cancers.

The 85 year old gent was "over the moon" with delight and everyone who knew him was utterly amazed at his transformation into normality. So much so that they got the Bexhill Observer to visit him at his warden care residence in Bexhill. The Observer gave me a front page spread on 29th December 1988. Even then, the medical people tried to prevent its publication.

From the resultant publicity, I had sugar farmers from Queensland Australia where almost every other one has skin cancer due to white men working all day in temperatures of 120 F in the sugar cane fields.   Irrespective of what type of skin cancer they had, they soon 'lost it' with my celandine lotion, including the deadly malignant melanoma.

One rather hilarious thing about Mr Brewster's case was that after I had spent a month patiently daily painting the celandine lotion on his hideous facial, head and hand cancers until finally he was totally clear, overcome with joy the dear old chap gave me a fiver for my trouble!   Of course £5 was more than a week's wages when he was a young man and I expect he tended to dwell in the past. However, as far as I was concerned, nothing else mattered other than beating his awful problem and the exhilaration I got from this. When you think scientists talk about many years necessary in research for almost any given disease, while I crack the very worst and think I'm dragging my feet if I take longer than three weeks!

Obviously, I get sceptics who try to rubbish me and some have said (mainly doctors), "how can you prove that drug induced Candida can mask out medicinal effects?" "Well", I replied, "whenever I am referred, patients who are very ill under orthodox treatment, without exception they are all initially untreatable" (even to the very doctors they were under and hence why they came to me). Now how could this be if it was not for medicinal masking by Candida for there is absolutely no other explanation for neither mine or doctors' medicine can work initially. So my very first job with a new very ill patient is to knock out their massive drug induced population of Candida that needs the essential anti-candida diet to weaken this devilish parasitic fungus, and then in its weakened state annihilate it with encapsulated wormwood. Within days of this happening the patient becomes as treatable as almost any other and within weeks (even less sometimes) these patients will be either in remission or well on the way to being so. This then is the proof absolute and until someone in authority takes this fact aboard, all the untouchables and world's very worst diseases will remain exactly as they have for years and to infinity.

The above facts are possibly the most important to bring about a vastly improved medical revolution. It will, however, be resisted vigorously by the pharma/medical network who will probably deny on the Good Book, if necessary, that their very drugs are the real cause of the medicinal masking factor and a whole list of untouchable diseases. The facts in above paragraphs would save countless patients suffering, not to mention many millions of pounds wasted as today in our NHS through not being able to treat effectively a lot of our very worst diseases.

CHAPTER 10

Summary of diseases and formulas

Now for a summary of the diseases which can be totally transformed and in some cases eliminated, or at least up to 100% relief remission given to cooperative patients aided by their doctors. The doctors have to be taught that the anti-candida diet is essential not only for all the terrible diseases mentioned but also to rid our land of the obese epidemic this diet would eliminate.

Lung Diseases

Some families have a genetic weakness to troublesome diseases and my family's weak point are lung diseases. My grandmother, father and me all suffered from bronchitis often for months at a time during the winter. Now as anyone knows who suffers in a similar way, there are really no effective orthodox remedies for lung disease and antibiotics often do not even touch severe bronchitis. Today with my lung Triple Alliance formula that saved my own life when I had severe bronchial asthma that brought me into alternative medicine in the first place, I never get bronchitis any more, even if I did, it would be knocked out in a couple of days. I assure my readers outside of my lung Triple Alliance formula there is no such medicine that can do that. So what lung diseases can it alleviate? Well **asthma and bronchitis**, the latter very quickly, the former slower but gives great relief. **Bronchiectasis**, this is often the advanced form of repeat attacks of bronchitis but is very much worse and sometimes fatal in bad cases. I have seen this supposed incurable disease completely removed by my lung Triple Alliance formula and quickly made better to remission where not. **Emphysema** is not an actual lung disease but lung destruction caused by something else i.e. smoking, fumes, dust, or in my case very severe asthma which can crush lung tissue. **Pneumonia** - I have personally had this disease knocked out in four days by the lung Triple Alliance formula. **Pleurisy** is inflammation of the lung lining and this needs antibiotics quickly and is very painful. So basically virtually any lung disease except pleurisy will be taken care of by the lung Triple Alliance.

Imagine what this wonderful formula could do against Cystic Fibrosis?

See letter here from Peggy Thorpe – following taking my lung Triple Alliance formula - all gone forever in a few weeks.

Very severe lung disease utterly annihilated by the lung Treble Alliance formula in liquid format

1993.

Five years ago, I was on my last
legs with Bronchitis, Pneumonia & Plurisy.
My Husband George, took me to see
Gerald Green, as ill as I was, I knew
I wanted some help. Gerald said
"I will make you feel better and in
Four weeks you will be cured".
George mixed the herbs up for me,
I took three wine glasses a day.
After five days I said to George.
"My tubes & Chest are clear and
I feel so much better." It is Four
years now that I have never had
Bronchitis, Pneumonia, or Plurisy again.
It is wonderfull, my greatest thanks
go to Gerald for curing me.
I would not be here now if it
wasnt for Gerald. Can I say more
            Peggy Thorpe

Gut Diseases

The gut Triple Alliance variation of above. This is easily the finest gut formula on earth and will remove or alleviate the very worst gut diseases on earth and will not be long about it either. The auto-immune disease orientated Crohn's disease and similar ulcerative-colitis are the two worst non-malignant gut diseases in the world and are well covered earlier in this book by this wonderful formula in both its normal gelatine and delayed release capsules which attack the ulceration and inflammation right in the epicentre of where these diseases attack at 100% strength with devastating effect against immunological flares common in newly referred patients.

Duodenal/Stomach Ulcers

Then there are both stomach and duodenal ulcers which I know from personal experience can be very painful and the sooner knocked out the better, as I suffered over seven years under orthodoxy, whereas with the gut Triple Alliance, my suffering was all over and done with in only four and a half weeks and gone forever. How? Well after a very long time in gut diseases, starting with me, as an experiment I tried the weakened wax walls of my Crohn's disease delayed release capsule necessary for it to release some seventeen feet down the small bowel right in the epicentre of where this disease attacks, activated by the digestive enzymes sent out in the duodenum (top of the small bowel). However, as I said, because of a poor output of digestive enzymes in auto-immune orientated Crohn's diseases patients the delayed release capsule has to have the wax weakened by adding solid sunflower oil in with bees wax, otherwise it would go straight through them unreleased and be useless.

So I had a "brain wave" and tried these Crohn's type weakened walled delayed release capsules on my duodenal ulcer. At my very first attempt it worked like a dream because when the delayed release capsule entered the duodenum and it was squirted with <u>normal</u> emulsifying digestive enzymes which break down fat molecules (and of course waxes and sunflower oil are exactly this) thus weakened, it released instantly right in the duodenum where the ulcer was quickly knocked out with the 100% full strength of the gut Triple Alliance formula. So that took care of the common duodenal ulcer and quickly too!

With a stomach ulcer there is no need to delay release because obviously the gut Triple Alliance formula in normal gelatine capsules will release the moment it falls into the stomach again right on the ulcer at 100% strength with again maximum quickest result possible.

Diverticulitis

Diverticulitis is a disease caused by eating white bread over much of a lifetime. Bran taken out of white bread grain holds twenty times its weight in water. However, our gut was evolved to digest wheat wholemeal with the bran and when wholemeal is ingested there was absolutely no trouble because the colon or large bowel recycles almost half of the water we either drink or eat in vegetables and fruit.

With all the bran in the bread as in wholemeal, the colon does not pull much water out of the bread waste because the bran absorbs twenty times its own weight in water so keeps the colon's contents soft and easy for the colon to move from right to left as it does all the time and it's never overworked. However, when white bread comes in (which our gut was not evolved for) the colon recycling could pull a great deal of water from the bread waste in the colon so making its contents very stiff, causing the poor colon to labour much harder than it should, so causing the little folds in the colon to become deeper and eventually inflamed. Those folds are called the diverticular and 'tis' in Latin means inflammation and hence the name of the disease diverticulitis which can vary from a mild condition to being absolutely life threatening. It is sadly an incurable disease (man made) but my gut Triple Alliance in both normal and a very special delayed release capsule covered in pure bees wax works well and quickly too.

The reason the diverticular delayed release capsules have this harder bees wax coating is because these patients usually have normal digestive enzymes (unlike for Crohn's patients) etc so to get the capsule to release at the end of the small bowel/start of the colon it needs this much stronger coating. Again on releasing these in the epicentre of where the disease attacks at 100% strength the Triple Alliance formula then swells up to 4 times the size of the capsule into an anti-inflammatory ball of gel that "paints" the colon wall as it passes through eliminating all inflammation very quickly and efficiently.

Usually the diverticular patient is relieved completely in three or four days but continues this treatment of taking 4 times a day normal Triple Alliance capsules plus two delayed release capsules making 6 all told for the first ten days and will then go into remission.

How long the remission will last is impossible to say for it may be weeks, months, or even years. But like the proverbial "bad penny" it will come back again because, as said, the disease is incurable. When it does return you hit it instantly and the patient may find they can knock out the attack with the normal Triple Alliance capsules, but if not use also the delayed release capsules. Eventually, the patient will become so well they (even former severe cases of diverticular disease) may only get one attack in a year or even less. It will however never be the devil it was prior to this treatment c/o this wonderful formula and the mechanics of the essential initial delayed release capsules.

Heart Burn

While on gut diseases and a very very common painful nuisance is 'heart burn'. While the actual stomach is well protected against being burnt by hydrochloric acid (there to turn your chewed up food into a sort of pre-digested soup called chyme) by a film of special mucus, your oesophagus connection from throat to the stomach has no such mucus protection so if the patient was to get a reflux from the stomach's contents (especially where an eddy caused by a hiatus hernia in the oesophagus is relevant) then it can be very painful and uncomfortable. I personally believe this could, in some cases, be the precursor of oesophageal cancer. However, it's simply got over by putting the highly compressed contents of a normal gut Triple Alliance capsule into a teacup and pouring in about a third of a teacup of hot water. Stir well and drink as hot as is comfortable and the heart burn will be gone in seconds, minutes at the outside with a possible "burp".

IBS

Irritable bowel syndrome causes a lot of grief and discomfort and the doctor will say "it's in no way serious". Yes to a point this is true but if the patient is say planning a holiday and the excitement causes them to cancel the holiday arrangements because it triggers off the pain and discomfort that are very real, this to a degree is seriously affecting their lives. The causes are many but the most common is in the nervous system to the colon which causes it to sometimes (i.e. when a patient is upset or excited etc.) contort instead of the usual rhythmic push of the large bowel contents eternally from right to left. This causes the contents perhaps to remain too long in one place and they then tend to ferment causing gas that pressurises the colon causing colic pain and discomfort. It causes so much misery yet many remedies are ineffective.

One of the best is my MS formula because the actual carrier of the immune ingredient are antispasmodics relative to spasms suffered by MS sufferers, but they obviously don't need the immune ingredient as IBS as it's called is not an auto-immune disease. This works brilliantly on 50% of IBS sufferers and the gut Triple Alliance formula works on 20% but in theory it should not - but does. So this covers 70% of all IBS sufferers.

I send out a trial of each as the patient has a 70% chance of finding their salvation. The other 30% are usually where the patient has dietary allergens that actually trigger the symptoms on ingestion, these most likely being orientated by Candida. Then it's obviously a case of trial and error in a dietary regime whereby the patient cuts out a dietary item every week re suspect items and when the patient suddenly gets better on an exclusion of an item, then it must be the allergen or one of them. So get rid of it and replace with any sensible alternative that doesn't contain sugar, yeast or cows' milk or its products loved by our enemy Candida. End of problem.

This shows just how complex IBS really is and why so few practitioners are successful with it. In a booklet I wrote on gut diseases twenty-five years ago I called it, "IBS the 'Enigma Variations' " which sums it up. I cannot think of a situation where the gut Triple Alliance formula could not be used against any gut disease (except malignant) and it is so very safe and gentle it can be used on tots and babies where it has been my privilege to save their lives by asking the mothers to give the gut Triple Alliance formula in a baby's feeding bottle using a larger than usual hole in the teat so that the warmed contents of the gel-like liquid mixture goes easily through.

For seriously ill babies I use the usual Triple Alliance formula but with a little extra slippery elm in it. The beauty of this when made up into a liquid by bringing it to a boil (so sterilising it), but also with the extra slippery elm in it gels up better and mother can use an egg whisk to ensure no lumps block up the hole in the teat. The extra slippery elm is also very nutritive so helping a possibly emaciated and very ill baby in more than one way. You may know the pH scale of relative alkalinity and acidity, well before boiling to make up this liquid format of the gut Triple Alliance formula for babies and tots the relative pH value is neutral. However, when it boils to get the anti-inflammatory gel effect it changes to slightly alkaline, which is useful to correct excess acidity in infants and also adult patients. This concludes gut diseases.

Helping patients to conceive – 'legally'!!

With diseases as vicious and violent as Crohn's and ulcerative colitis, patients can have difficulty in conceiving. Indeed the latter is applicable in a number of other auto immune diseases where not having children can be a heart wrenching factor in a partnership already with its difficulties.

So seeing such ladies in distress to a point of tears, I felt it my job to read up on the subject of conception. I read up just about everything and just one herb stood out as possibly what I was looking for to help IBD patients. It goes under two names, one being false unicorn and the other helonias root. It thins down the mucous in the fallopian tubes which makes the sperms journey to conception easier. In addition to that, believe it or not, it has the beneficial side effect of preventing miscarriages.

I used it on a young lady Crohn's sufferer and she conceived within a few weeks and a fine healthy son was born. Everyone was naturally delighted, as was I, achieving another first. As time when on, word spread and more of my patients opted for this herb and to date I have witnessed nine 'happy events' (it working superbly most times). Some of the ladies were on IVF when I treated them and some were not – it did not seem to make a difference. The ladies and I were delighted as all the babies were normal healthy ones but the very strange thing was they were all boys!

My latest lady Jo was desperate, having spent thousands of pounds on IVF treatment to no avail. Within weeks of me treating her, in conjunction with IVF, she was able to conceive and again a fine healthy baby was born and no points are gained for guessing what sex it was! Yes a beautiful healthy boy called Rhys. Five years past and Jo wanted another baby for Rhys to grow up with so Jo said "I'll give your treatment a miss this time because I would love to have a girl so I'll go back to just IVF treatment again". I said to her it was perfectly understandable and best of luck.

Nearly two expensive IVF years past with again no success and when Jo came for her gut Triple Alliance capsules which had held her ulcerative-colitis in remission for over twelve years, she said what does it matter if Rhys does have a brother to grow up with even though she would have preferred a girl. So I gave Jo the helonias root tincture (again to be used in conjunction with IVF) and she soon conceived and had a normal pregnancy – except her tummy seemed to be growing rather fast. A scan at the hospital confirmed for me another first, namely twins and joy of joys a boy and a girl - which to all of us was the proverbial 'icing on the cake'!

I have to say I have absolutely no idea why all the babies prior to this were boys, while who is to say that by Jo having twins this may have been the only way to break this sequence? Whatever, it was a splendid end to a wonderful sequence of events.

Cardiovascular Disease

Possibly the greatest killer is coronary disease where the arteries on the actual heart block up or narrow that supplies the heart muscle with blood and oxygen necessary for its efficiency. Needless to say, if it became completely blocked the heart pump would stop and the patient naturally would be dead. As I mentioned earlier in this book, this in 80% of patients is completely unnecessary when you use the herbal chilli/cayenne red pepper "Dino Rod" capsule to clear out the deposits that clog not only the coronary artery but the whole vascular system.

<u>Claudication</u>

Exactly the same "Dino Rod" treatment completely does away with common claudication which can cause terrible suffering and sometimes limbs have to be amputated if the blood and oxygen supply to the legs is cut off by blocked arteries. Warnings are aching limbs which tire easily when walking. This problem can easily be sorted out or alleviated and all the unnecessary suffering of this and associated varicose ulcers.

Under cardio-vascular disease comes **high blood pressure** which kills and maims thousands unnecessarily relative to strokes. There are two types of stroke i.e. namely where through high blood pressure causes a "blow-out" in the brain flooding it with blood, this being the most dangerous as it's very difficult to stop the bleeding. The other type of stroke is caused by clots of blood blocking the veins in the brain. What does not get blood and oxygen discontinues to function and the brain is damaged. Patients who take red pepper capsules have much less chance of this happening, but orthodoxy has clot busting drugs which I had after an operation c/o deep vein thrombosis and it was successful. Who says I never praise the doctors!! but have to say they caused the DVT c/o the operation in the first place but was not really their fault.

Red pepper helps beyond belief a host of problems, especially with middle aged and elderly. The latter would, of course, have to be supervised unless they were 100% in charge of their minds c/o the possibility mentioned above which, as said, need not be with care and commonsense. Red pepper can also be added to a foot bath where it most certainly helps the **circulation,** say a dessertspoonful in a bowl of warm water. It works via osmosis i.e. goes through the skin to the capillaries increasing circulation and inducing warmth and a glowing feel to the feet and very worthwhile especially in circulatory problems like **Raynaud's disease.**

One highly beneficial side-effect of chilli pepper is that it vastly improves circulation all over the body having cleared out the whole vascular system. Because of this everything is well supplied with blood and oxygen including the synovial glands that supply all of our joints and tendon sheaths with a lubricating fluid and this obviously alleviates arthritis and rheumatism. Add to this where relevant glucosamine from health shops and you may well have a new lease of life free from so many problems, or at least greatly alleviated.

In addition to yet another wonderful medicine is Hawthorn which can do so much for a failing heart in the elderly. It assists coronary disease by having a bradycardic effect on the myocardium (strengthens the heart muscle) often damaged in coronary disease and will slow down a racing heart beat. Blood pressure itself is well covered especially the very severe malignant type handed down to me by my mother. This is taken care of with the wonderful herb, barberry, which can knock off a hundred degrees on the mercury scale in an hour which no machine on earth can do except barberry and is <u>useful only in very severe blood pressure like I was subjected to</u>. It could save many lives and intense misery relative to strokes caused by very high blood pressure that orthodox medicine cannot, simply because it is not powerful enough in these extreme cases.

So I've covered all gut, lung and vascular disease not to mention the "untouchables" in the auto-immune group, also cancer and leukaemia and I never pick easy to treat patients. The only type I treat are the right off the scale of severity who have been written off by their doctors and are way beyond their help. They are not that difficult especially with the ladies who will not, as a rule, put a glass of beer before their very lives like so many men will and stick rigidly to the diet.

CHAPTER 11

General Remedies

Kidney stones

Kidney stones can cause intense pain and can often result in operations to remove them, sometimes causing damage to these vital organs. Obviously it is far and away better to dissolve them in the kidneys with another wonder herb called parsley piert which cannot be given in capsule format but as a liquid sherry glass dose 4 x day spaced throughout the day. Kidney stones seem as hard as 'stones' yet when this wonderful herb is digested, it quickly reacts on these hard stones and shatters them.

The only side effect is pain sometimes when passing water, and several of my male patients have said to me they could hear the fragmented bits of former stone clinking on the porcelain urinal after only a few days treatment, showing how effective the parsley piert herb is.

To make up the liquid medicine is easy. Get a <u>wide necked </u>soup flask – put in ¾ ounce (approx. 23 grams) of parsley piert herb which, being light in weight, is a fair amount. Fill the flask with very hot water (being two minutes off the boil). Replace the top and leave for approximately twenty minutes. It will then be drawn (extracted) in the water so pour initially through a flour sieve, pressing out with a saucer most of the liquid in the herb. When this is done, finally sieve the liquid through a tea-strainer and to the liquid make it up with cold water to one and a quarter pints (just over 700 ml). This equals eight sherry glasses which if taken at 4 x a day lasts two days (its shelf life will be no more than that). Then simply make up another batch until you have completed two weeks treatment and by then your kidneys should be clear of all stones.

I have found out in practice that kidney stones are more common in males and, strange as it may seem, patients who suffer this problem repeatedly seem to lose calcium from their bones and then it forms stones in the kidneys. I cannot stop this completely but suggest they take a boron supplement (obtained from health shops) to help prevent possible osteoporosis. However, I most certainly can prevent the stones forming again by simply dissolving forming stones at sand size particles by making up the parsley piert herb liquid every two months for just two days – and you will not have them form again.

If you think this wonderful treatment is something new, think again, because in the days of Queen Elizabeth I, women sold the parsley piert herb in Cheapside London shouting their wares from the streets calling it parsley break stone.

Gall Stones

Myra Finlay, the Australian lady who helped me with publicity to crack multiple sclerosis in Australia in 1996 and mentioned earlier in this book, rang me to say she was in absolute agony with gall stones and her consultant correctly said to her that there was no herb that would dissolve gall stones like there is for kidney stones and she must have an operation to remove them. However, Myra was none too keen to have the operation, fearful not so much of the risk of the operation, but what she might 'pick up' in the way of super bugs that make almost everyone worry these days and very understandably. She therefore asked me if I could help her.

I advised her there was a way of getting rid of her gall stones but she would have to be brave and there could be some pain (but she was in great pain anyway) and it would take five hours laying on her left-hand side on a sofa or bed while drinking one and a quarter litres of virgin olive oil and lemon juice. It sounds a bit drastic but it worked brilliantly and naturally Myra was absolutely delighted and her consultant was utterly amazed when the hospital scan showed that all Myra's multiple stones were gone!

What happens is that by drinking so much olive oil, laced with lemon juice (which helps prevent nausea) it causes the liver and bile duct to go into 'over-drive' and then forces the actual stones out of the neck of the gall bladder. This is exactly what happened to Myra laying on her left-hand side which makes the ejection of the stones easier.

Here is an extract from the letter she wrote me following this success:

"Dear Gerald
Thank you so much for your information in my time of need re the painful gall stone/bladder problem. It worked superbly and joy of joys it negated surgery. My specialist has said rather patronizingly "there is nothing in alternative medicine that will dissolve gall stones" so he had booked me for surgery. No one was more surprised than him when I told him that I had got rid of all my stones and he did not believe me. You can imagine the surgeon's amazement when

an MRI scan proved I was totally clear of the gall stones shown on my initial scan!"

MF

As said, although the gall stones could not be dissolved, the above method blasted the stones out of the bladder by making the liver go into 'over-drive.' The stones then travel down the bile duct, lubricated by the olive oil, into the duodenum and then through the bowel system and out.

Not everyone would be brave enough to go through the above regime, but it does away with the risks of surgery, infections etc and Myra was more than happy with the result.

More General Remedies

For healing simple wounds then a tincture made from the herb, St Johns Wort, is unbeatable when diluted (also called hypericum perforatum). **Ear infections** can be quickly eliminated by taking Echinacea capsules to boost the immune system and attack them from within, while golden seal drops used from a dropper are used externally and will eliminate the problem very quickly.

Indeed any infection as mentioned or **abscess**, the simple rule is to attack it from within by boosting the immune system with Echinacea and then using either St. Johns Wort diluted tincture, or if in the eyes golden seal drops diluted to suit your eyes. Rule of thumb is it should be a clear golden colour and should not smart the eyes and, if it does, dilute until comfortable.

Another rather unpleasant problem is **mouth ulcers**, especially with false teeth. A very simple remedy that usually works like lightning is live yoghurt, or a health drink I make up called Kefir. Simply when going to bed fill the mouth with live yoghurt so it goes underneath the false teeth plate, if relevant, then swallow the excess and then go to sleep and the good bugs in it will soon eliminate the ulcers quickly. If you don't like yoghurt then use sage tea exactly as above and again it will make short work of any ulcers. It must be live yoghurt as when mixed with fruit juice it won't work.

CHAPTER 12

<u>Chemicals v Organic</u>

Finally, I would like to have a word on our food and chemical additives that may procreate so much of the misery written about in this book. Doctors, as you may have noticed, hardly ever criticise the use of chemicals in our food chain. However, I would say, eat and drink organic produced food that's free of these nasty chemicals. Oh yes, men from the ministry tell us it's "absolutely safe" to ingest organo-phosphorous in small amounts on most inorganic food, not to mention battery chicken stuffed with antibiotics to try and get over the deplorable conditions these poor creatures suffer under.

Think about the people born with either a genetic weakness to, or a fragility in their immune systems that I am absolutely certain orientate to the awful auto-immune diseases mentioned in my book. Also, if you continue to ingest the chemicals mentioned and some not, plus antibiotics in so many of the farm animals we eat, it must weaken your constitution, not to mention by ingesting antibiotics, bad bugs get used to them. So if then you get a life threatening infection, antibiotics may not be effective because they are very similar to those used on farm animals.

As you saw at the front of this book, Jo Wood was delighted to write the foreword. Nearly twenty years ago it was my pleasure to help Jo, wife of "Rolling Stone" Ronnie with a serious problem and I converted Jo to organic food that helped her and her family, very well portrayed in her book "Naturally" ISBN 9780283070419. In her first chapter Jo calls it appropriately "Finding Shangri-La" the name of my house, bless her. Her book tells of the really great advantages of eating and drinking healthily with many fine recipes. Yes, I know inorganic food is cheaper but you must ask yourself do you want to run the risk for your family, especially with seemingly a new super bug each year.

The Way Ahead

I hope this book has given you a good insight into the power of herbal remedies used with applied immunology and the essential diets against the "untouchable diseases". By and large I personally do not treat trivial health problems and just tell people how to get over, whatever, easily by using health shop products.

Going forward, I would love to see so much improvement in the world's worst diseases c/o the pioneering work portrayed in my book and for which orthodox medicine can often find little relief for. I have tried to teach a few others my work, but as you can imagine, some parts of it are rather complex and well beyond the comprehension of most lay people. However, over the years, I have taught a local lady to me Karin Taylor who has been able to understand my work and make up my remedies exactly as I have. She would like to continue my work after my life as retirement is not an option for me.

I will continue to the best of my ability 'til my time comes because what gives me a real buzz is to take on someone with a truly vicious deadly disease and give them up to 100% relief remission in double quick time and that does not cost the earth!

GERALD GREEN
Shangrila, 53 Downlands Close
Bexhill-on-Sea,
East Sussex,
TN39 3PP, ENGLAND
Telephone: 01424 218683

Chapter 13

LETTERS

I have hundreds and hundreds of thank you letters and progress charts, and it gives me great pleasure to end this book by sharing some of these with you.

N.B. The letters and charts / documents in the body of this book were scanned from the originals to enable them to be included as part of the book. Consequently, some of them are not as legible as the originals which can be viewed by appointment.

Dear Mr Green

As a bit of a low down on myself here goes:
I am 27, the doctors found out that I have Crohnes at the age of 18. I actually contracted it about the age of 12 but it took years of various types of medication (which didn't work) (and a doctor telling me it was all in my head) and two collapses before they finally did the tests to find out what I had.
Since then I have been on Prednisalone almost constantly and I have had to have two operations. I now only have 15cm of large bowel left and 8 foot of small bowel. I can't afford to loose any more. Also as an added complication I have lost over 35% of my bone density in my hips and spine especially, due to the steroids. I am willing to try anything new and I am already trying to figure out some nice things to eat if you take away Sweets, biscuits, marmite, cheese etc. (all my favourites). I really don't want to have to go through another op.p. like the last one.
Thank you for the work you are doing for people like me. I look forward to hearing from you soon.

Yours sincerely

Caroline A

SEE ATTACHED PROGRESS CHART

GG

If proof was needed of the terrible vagaries of orthodox treatment, here is the classic example of where the drugs, c/o induced Candida sent this formally awful case of Crohn's in a 27 year old patient, out of control leading to dreadful maiming surgery. Note too the diabolical side effects of long term steroid use causing a 35% loss of bone density, leaving this young lady wide open to crippling osteoporosis.

MONITORING CHART for CROHN'S and ULCERATIVE COLITIS

DAY/ DATE	0	Week 1	Week 2	Week 3	Week 4
Symptoms					
Pain / Colic	S	S\M	SL	SL	Gone
Bleeding	N\A				
Number of bowel movements daily	10-15	7-10	7-10	5-7	3-5
Fistulas	?				
Number of operations prior to herbal / dietary treatment. Please state which.	2 operations had 2½ foot of bowel removed (8 foot small bowel left + 15cm large)				
Bowel narrowing	S	S\M	SL	SL	None
Nausea and sickness	S	SL	Gone	Gone	Gone
Emaciation and weight loss	S	S\M	SL	SL	Gaining
Associated arthritis	m	m	m	SL	None
Associated anaemia	m	m	SL	Gone	Gone
Bloating or distension	m	SL	Gone	Gone	Gone
Constipation					
Proctitis					
Stools formed as opposed to diarrhoea	Never			SL	
Areas affected but not normally associated by IBD	Bone density down by 35% Eyesight affected (GG CAUSED BY STEROIDS)				
Drugs taken, please state;	Prednisolone, Imodium				
Relief given	M	M	lots	Relief 80	R 85%
Any other symptoms; please state.	All the side effects				
General opinion of herbal v drug treatment	So much better. No side effects				
What was the response from your gastroenterologist upon embarking on this treatment?	A pat on the head - try it if i want to but it wont work.				

Please indicate severity of symptoms prior to treatment in column O, for example;
S = SEVERE M = MODERATE SL = SLIGHT
Using this code, continue through the weeks, showing relief or lack of it and write the word GONE where relative.
Week O is the start of treatment, please indicate whether or not symptoms are slight, moderate or severe.

Name	CAROLINE A
Address	
Telephone Number	
Comments;	Since going on the diet + taking the herbal tablets my life has gone from being unbearable to enjoyable. Thankyou! I have my life back.

GERALD GREEN
MEDICAL HERBALIST
& IMMUNOLOGIST
Tel. Bexhill 218443 (Afternoon)

Unusual Crohn's case with associated immunelogical orientated severe arthritis & anaemia. Indeed so severe was the arthritis in this twenty year old patient, her hands had nodules on them like an eighty year old arthritic. Imagine the misery of Crohn's, plus when it flared, so did Erica's arthritis & anaemia. With my Triple Alliance capsules & essential diets, her misery symptom wise is ended in total remission for a life free of terrible suffering, surgery, drugs and their side effects.

MONITORING CHART for CROHN'S and ULCERATIVE COLITIS

DAY/DATE 3rd February, '97	0	Week 1	Week 2	Week 3	Week 4
Symptoms					
Pain / Colic	SL		GONE		
Bleeding	SL			GONE	
Number of bowel movements daily	4/5	GONE			
Fistulas	N/A				
Number of operations prior to herbal / dietary treatment. Please state which.	N/A				
Bowel narrowing	N/A				
Nausea and sickness	M	GONE			
Emaciation and weight loss	S	(Starting gaining weight after 12 weeks)			
Associated arthritis	M	(Gone after 14 weeks)			
Associated anaemia	M	(Gone after 7 weeks)			
Bloating or distension	SL				GONE
Drugs taken, please state;	Short course of Prednisolone (10 days). Asacol tablets every day - no longer required.				
Relief given	Stopped diarrhoea, and all other symptoms				
Constipation	M	GONE			
Stools formed as opposed to diarrhoea	M				GONE
Areas affected but not normally associated by IBD : i.e. Proctitis	N/A				
Any other symptoms; please state.	(piles, cramp, sweats, numbness, swollen feet) GONE				
General opinion of herbal v drug treatment	Herbal much better - no horrid side effects				
What was the response from your gastroenterologist upon embarking on this treatment?	GP. was sympathetic with me trying your treatment and was glad I was getting better - have not seen hospital specialist since I have been on your treatment				

Please indicate severity of symptoms prior to treatment in column O, for example;
S = SEVERE   M = MODERATE   SL = SLIGHT
Using this code, continue through the weeks, showing relief or lack of it and write the word GONE where relative.
Week O is the start of treatment, please indicate whether or not symptoms are slight, moderate or severe.

Name	ERICA
Address	
Telephone Number	
Comments;	I now feel much healthier. It's such a relief to be 'normal' again. Many thanks
	ENC

4th May 1998

Dear Mr Green,

I wanted to write to thank you for your assistance since we began using your Herbal treatments in conjunction with the 'anti-candida' and elimination diet.

The herbal treatment and diets relieved symptoms of acute diarrhoea bowel spasms, fainting nausea general pallour and feeling unwell within 48 hours.

I couldn't believe how much better I felt. It is only since following your regime I have come to realise how much pain I was experiencing daily. Now I can go out without fear of accidents.

I'm no longer reliant on drugs which are unpleasant to take with lists of side effects and poor long term effect.

Your treatment is effective and has NO side effects

I worked in a hospital for some time and have seen the tragic outcome for some IBD patients who eventually have to rely on butcher-like surgery Which still is not curative but simply adds to their suffering and embarrassment. I can wholeheartedly recommend your remedies to anyone and will be glad to share my experiences of ulcerative collitis and your treatment and diet. Please let me know if I can be of assistance in the future.

Yours sincerely

K.H Newell.

P.S. As I am feeding my baby still it is great to know I can experience 100% relief from U.C. symptoms without any harmful drugs being passed through my milk to the baby!

136

MS TREATMENT MONITORING CHART

DAY/ DATE	0	Week 1	Week 2	Week 3	Week 4
Symptoms					
DOUBLE VISION/OPTIC NEURITIS					
~~SLURRED SPEECH~~ DIFFICULTY IN SWALLOWING	OCC	GONE	GONE	GONE	GONE
JAW UNABLE TO OPEN FULLY					
NUMB MOUTH/TONGUE/GUMS					
NUMB SCALP/FACE	OCC	GONE	GONE	GONE	GONE
NUMB ~~STOMACH~~ ACROSS ABDOMIN	S	S	S	GONE	GONE
NUMB LEFT ARM					
DIZZINESS	M	SL	SL	GONE	GONE
~~WEAKNESS~~ CRAWLING SENSATION RIGHT SIDE AND BACK	SL	SL	SL	GONE	GONE
LOSS OF BALANCE	M	M	M	GONE	GONE
EXTREME FATIGUE					
HEAVINESS IN RIGHT ARM	SL	SL	GONE	GONE	GONE
HEAVINESS IN LEFT ARM					
HEAVINESS IN RIGHT LEG	S	M	M	M	M
PAIN ~~WEAKNESS~~ IN LEFT ~~LEG~~ KNEE	S	S	S	GONE	GONE
WEAKNESS IN RIGHT HAND	SL	SL	GONE	GONE	GONE
WEAKNESS IN LEFT HAND					
VERTIGO					
BLADDER INCONTINENCE	S	SL	GONE	GONE	GONE
BOWEL INCONTINENCE					
CONSTIPATION	SL	GONE	GONE	GONE	GONE
SPASM IN LEGS	M	M	SL	SL	SL
SPASMS IN ARMS					
Feet ~~LIMBS~~ EXTREMELY COLD	SL	SL	SL	GONE	GONE
LIMBS EXTREMELY HOT					
SENSITIVE TO CHEMICALS					
PINS AND NEEDLES HANDS & FEET.	SL	SL	SL	SL	GONE
MIGRAINE					
EMOTIONAL PROBLEMS					
CO-ORDINATION	M	SL	SL	SL	GONE
SEXUAL DYSFUNCTION					
PAIN	M	SL	GONE	GONE	GONE

Please underline if you have ; REMITTING MS / PROGRESSIVE MS
Please indicate severity of symptoms prior to treatment in column O, for example;
S = SEVERE   M = MODERATE   SL = SLIGHT   OCC - OCCAISIONALLY
Using this code, continue through the weeks, showing relief or lack of it and write the word GONE
where relative.

Name	LYNNE F
Address	
Telephone Number	
Comments;	DELIGHTED + IMPRESSED LIKE A MIRACLE

137

GERALD GREEN
MEDICAL HERBALIST
& IRIDOLOGIST
Tel & 6201 01601 (Ryburn-)

Ref. Jill

Former nursing Sister was so severely disabled by MS, she was hardly able to use a wheelchair. Within just four weeks of using my unique MS formula and dietary regime, Jill is able to walk unaided with most of her awful symptoms gone or going.

MS TREATMENT MONITORING CHART

DAY/ DATE 15 . 2 . 00	0	Week 1	Week 2	Week 3	Week 4
Symptoms					
DOUBLE VISION/OPTIC NEURITIS					
SLURRED SPEECH	M	SL	SL	SL	SL
JAW UNABLE TO OPEN FULLY					
NUMB MOUTH/TONGUE/GUMS					
NUMB SCALP/FACE					
NUMB RIGHT ARM					
NUMB LEFT ARM					
DIZZINESS					
WEAKNESS	S	SL	SL	SL	gone
LOSS OF BALANCE	S	SL	SL	SL	SL
EXTREME FATIGUE	M	M	M	M/SL	SL
HEAVINESS IN RIGHT ARM	S	gone	gone	gone	gone
HEAVINESS IN LEFT ARM	S	M	SL	SL	SL
HEAVINESS IN RIGHT LEG	S	M	SL	SL	SL
HEAVINESS IN LEFT LEG					gone
WEAKNESS IN RIGHT HAND					
WEAKNESS IN LEFT HAND	SL	—	SL	SL	gone
VERTIGO					
BLADDER INCONTINENCE	M	SL	SL	gone	gone
BOWEL INCONTINENCE					
CONSTIPATION	SL	SL	SL	SL	SL
SPASM IN LEGS					
SPASMS IN ARMS					
LIMBS EXTREMELY COLD	M	M	M	M/SL	SL
LIMBS EXTREMELY HOT					
SENSITIVE TO CHEMICALS					
PINS AND NEEDLES					
MIGRAINE					
EMOTIONAL PROBLEMS					
CO-ORDINATION	M	SL	SL	SL	V/SL
SEXUAL DYSFUNCTION					
PAIN					

Please underline if you have ; REMITTING MS / PROGRESSIVE MS
Please indicate severity of symptoms prior to treatment in column O, for example;
S = SEVERE   M = MODERATE   SL = SLIGHT
Using this code, continue through the weeks, showing relief or lack of it and write the word GONE where relative.

Name	JILL W
Address	
Telephone Number	
Comments;	I cant believe i'm so well alredy

99 Jills writing

Four weeks ago Jill was hardly able to use a wheelchair and had major toiletary problems. Now she can walk short distances unaided. With more confidence and exercise I am sure she will do even better.

99 Jills dad

138

GERALD GREEN
MEDICAL HERBALIST
& IRIDOLOGIST
[illegible]

Ref Margaret

Margaret had lain paralytic for eight long years with about as severe as MS gets. Yet within a month on my unique MS capsules, & dietary regime, she is taking her first steps, with most of her terrible symptoms gone or going.

MS TREATMENT MONITORING CHART

DAY/ DATE	0	Week 1	Week 2	Week 3	Week 4
Symptoms 1 - 1 - 00					
DOUBLE VISION/OPTIC NEURITIS					
SLURRED SPEECH					
JAW UNABLE TO OPEN FULLY					
NUMB MOUTH/TONGUE/GUMS					
NUMB SCALP/FACE					
NUMB RIGHT ~~ARM~~ HAND	S	M	M	SL	SL
NUMB LEFT ~~ARM~~ HAND	S	S	S	S	M
DIZZINESS					
WEAKNESS					
LOSS OF BALANCE	S	S	S	M	M
EXTREME FATIGUE	SL	SL	GONE	GONE	GONE
HEAVINESS IN RIGHT ARM					
HEAVINESS IN LEFT ARM					
HEAVINESS IN RIGHT LEG	S	S	M	M	M
HEAVINESS IN LEFT LEG	S	S	S	S	M
WEAKNESS IN RIGHT HAND					
WEAKNESS IN LEFT HAND					
VERTIGO					
BLADDER INCONTINENCE					
BOWEL INCONTINENCE					
CONSTIPATION	S	SL	GONE	GONE	GONE
SPASM IN LEGS	M	SL	SL	GONE	GONE
SPASMS IN ARMS					
~~LIMBS~~ FEET EXTREMELY COLD	SL	GONE	GONE	GONE	GONE
LIMBS EXTREMELY HOT					
SENSITIVE TO CHEMICALS					
HALITOSIS (BAD BREATH)					
MIGRAINE					
EMOTIONAL PROBLEMS	M	GONE	GONE	GONE	GONE
CO-ORDINATION					
SEXUAL DYSFUNCTION					
PAIN	S	GONE	GONE	GONE	GONE

FEET

Please underline if you have ; REMITTING MS / PROGRESSIVE MS
Please indicate severity of symptoms prior to treatment in column O, for example;
S = SEVERE   M = MODERATE   SL = SLIGHT
Using this code, continue through the weeks, showing relief or lack of it and write the word GONE where relative.

Name	MARGARET P
Address	

I would like to emphasise that I cannot get fantastic results like this so quickly every time. If an MS patient has been on drugs, medicinal masking may prevent my unique MS formula working for up to 8-9 weeks. This letter shows the advantage of getting rid of the medicinal masking/immune trigger allergens from the diet first ie anti-candida and gluten exclusion diets (essential).

(GG)

7 March 1996

Dear Mr Green,

I respond to your invitation to let you know of any improvements I have noticed in the week since your MS medication arrived. I have been taking the capsules as instructed and have adopted your gluten-free anti-Candida diet since I phoned you several weeks ago. I list the improvements in the order I have experienced them

Better bladder control

Ability to stand from sitting without resorting to any form of support while doing so.

Ability to stand in shower, again without support.

Walking better with the walker.

Walking better when moving around the supp-orting walls without the walker.

Not using the walker sometimes when moving around the house, using a walking stick instead.

The swelling in my feet has considerably lessened and I have lost weight also, probably due to decreased water retention.

My eyesight has improved to the extent that I can often thread a needle at the first attempt.

Rest of letter non-relevant except thanks Signed Gwen C

GG When Gwen's muscles are built up, in 6 weeks or so, she will walk well again

140

Gerald Green
Shangri-La
53 Downlands Close
Bexhill-on-Sea
East Sussex
TN39 3PP

30 November 2005

Dear Gerald

As per our conversation recently, regarding the possibilities that I have systemic Candida. I have a life long history of exposure to anti-biotic treatments. Owing to a diagnosis of Pelvic Inflammatory Disease. I now constantly feel unwell and suffer from nausea constantly, have a poor appetite and extreme tiredness. Crave sugary drinks, larger, and wine (even though the latter makes me gag). I am now suffering bouts of headaches, fever, and vomiting. I cannot go on like this. Therefore, I am willing to try a trial course of the wormwood treatment you mentioned and anything else that may help me to feel better.

Gerald you have helped so many in my family that I have the utmost belief in your ability to heal. Thank you again for helping my son Dominick. His tutors believe he will be a great performer on the West End stage. All because of you. Please show this letter to anyone you wish and give him or her my phone number should they wish to ask questions.

Gerald I hate to ask this awful question, but should anything happen to you what will happen to your amazing healing tools? It would be a sin to humanity should it all be lost. I hope you do not mind me asking that question.

Yours sincerely

Rochelle C

[signature]

Rochelle's mother suffered from ulcerative colitis, her brother from Crohn's disease while her son Dominick had at the time a mystery illness that attacked his joints and muscles.   Because of the genetic link in the family I recognised it as another auto-immune disease fairly quickly – systemic lupus – the most deadly of all auto-immune diseases.

All of the above former sufferers now live in 100% relief remission.   Now young Dominick can continue his dancing career.

(GG)

Gerald Green Esq
Shangrila
53 Downlands Road
Bexhill-on-Sea
East Sussex
TN39 3PP

26th September 2003

Dear Mr Green

It is difficult, nay, impossible, for me to express my deep appreciation for your invaluable help, patience, and support, since my diagnosis with locally advanced cancer of the prostate.

I began my treatment on the 24th August, which consists of a mixture of hormone and blood pressure tablets, together with the herbs you have prescribed, a variety of supplements, and a strictly controlled diet, as per your guidelines.

When I was diagnosed my PSA reading was 22. Yesterday, from the blood sample taken 30 days after I began this regime my PSA reading is 1.4 (Yes one point four!!) *GG A few weeks later it was nil*

Whilst I expected that I would be some way towards the goal of eradicating this deadly threat to my well being, I am overjoyed that such an incredible result has been achieved in such a short space of time.

The diet is difficult to follow, but when one considers the benefits-reduced weight-lowered cholesterol-increased energy-and above all, the reward of conquering my life-threatening cancer, I realise that the odd bar of chocolate or glass of wine is really not so important

With renewed thanks!

Yours sincerely

Robert N.W

Robert N W

ITP = **Idiopathic Thrombocytopenic Purpura (low platelet count). This and Sarcoidosis (inflammation that produces tiny lumps of cells in various organs in the body) are both auto immune diseases. My immune ingredient in the Triple Alliance medicine knocks out the whole lot. Diet alone (anti candida) put up Katy's blood count before she received my medicine. Katy did not need the splenectomy after my treatment as her condition had improved so much.**

(GG)

Mr Gerald Green
"Shangrila"
53 Downlands Close
Bexhill-On-Sea
East Sussex
TN39 3PP

Dear Mr Green

Thank you again for your time and help you gave me on the telephone last night.

I have suffered from I.T.P for five years now, diabetes since March 9 this year. I am insulin dependant and have two injections per day. I have enclosed for your information a 'Patient Wise' description of I.T.P. Interestingly, this condition when pregnant can make your platelets go to normal out through the term of pregnancy but fall again once the baby has been born. (I am not pregnant!)

My platelet count is under ten at the moment, last count '8', normal is between 150-500. The doctors very much want me to have a splenectomy because my platelet count is so low. The weekend after next they want me to take four days worth of steroids called dexamethozone, 20mg a day (this is a high dosage over a short period - equivalent to 100mg of prednisolone). I cannot take prednisolone any more because it doesn't make any difference to my platelet count anymore.

Please could you forward to me with instructions so that hopefully I can prove to my Haematologist that someone does know about Auto Immune Diseases and even more so what causes them and how they can be treated. I am so pleased you haven't told me its caused by a Virus!

I thought I had better add, the day I was diagnosed with diabetes I was also diagnosed as having a conditions called Sarcoidosis, I don't know whether this is of any interest to you.

Thank you Mr Green.

Yours sincerely

Katy

Katy D

NB   I had a platelet count today and it was 62, perhaps the diet is making it better already.

6 weeks after Katy first wrote to me she sent me
this progress letter – Wow!

This also shows hope for those with Type I diabetes (GG)

Dear Mr Green,

Please find enclosed cheque for 'miracle
pills!' please can you send me some
more. A.S.A.P.

Mr Green, I am feeling the best I have
for ages, going on holiday abroad is
something I haven't been able to do for
2yrs. I have had I.T.P for 5yrs. I also
have been reducing my insulin, which
can't be a bad thing?

Thank you, Thank you, Thank you,

Love + Best wishes
from Katy X

The Sunday Mail heard of my work and some years ago published an article in their Sunday supplement magazine "You".
They tried and tested three alternative treatments – one of which was mine listed here:

"Tester – Judie, 48, shop manager, non-smoker
Problem: asthma, tiredness, irritable bowel syndrome.
My asthma started nearly ten years ago, after a bad chest infection.
I use a preventative inhaler called Becloforte plus Ventolin for
attacks. Every winter I get prolonged chest infections which
sometimes require steroid treatment. Gerald Green gave m
e three sets of herbal remedies: the Lung and Gut Triple Alliance
Formulas and a herbal remedy for IBS. I had to stay off dairy
products which was not easy as I love vanilla Ice cream and butter.
He also asked me to keep a food diary then exclude various items,
one at a time for two days and see if it made a difference to both
my asthma and my IBS.

I felt quite light-headed the first day I took the herbs but I've
been fine since. My asthma started improving after two days, in
the second week I had a bad throat bug but I took Ventolin only
once – a great improvement.

The diet was quite difficult to stick to. The best thing is that
I now eat more fresh food, rather than processed. After 4 weeks
the IBS had gone, I had no asthmatic symptoms and didn't need to
use my inhaler. Although I have finished taking the herbs, I'm still
off dairy products – it's hard work but very exciting to find a way
of controlling my asthma – I'm feeling very positive."

END